Women in Swedish Society

The Work, Health and Life Experiences of Women in Twentieth-century Sweden

Scandinavia and the Baltic – Transnational and International Challenges

Editor
Associate Professor Jason Lavery: Dept. of History, Oklahoma State University

Mission
This series primarily seeks scholarship in the disciplines known as 'Area Studies': history and the social sciences. It seeks scholarship that examines problems in the Nordic/Baltic region or a specific country that are transnational and or international in nature.

  This series will address many of the weaknesses of scholarship concerning Scandinavia available in English. First, it will broaden the work in English available concerning Scandinavia on issues that concern international audiences. Between the Vikings and the welfare state, there are few scholarly books that one can read about Scandinavia in English in history and the social sciences. It will aid those who teach Scandinavian history at the university level to provide their students with scholarship that will help them put Scandinavia in a larger perspective. Second, it will challenge the strong current trend in English-language area studies scholarship on Scandinavia that seeks to emphasize the uniqueness of Scandinavia in the global community. Third, it will provide opportunities for scholars to better integrate Scandinavia in the prevailing narratives in their respective fields.

Editorial Panel:
Nancy Wicker: Univ. of Mississippi
Eric Einhorn: Univ. of Massachusetts
Mary Hilson: University of London
Mikko Ketola: University of Helsinki

Women in Swedish Society

The Work, Health and Life Experiences of Women in Twentieth-century Sweden

Annika Forssén and Gunilla Carlstedt

Translated by Rochelle Wright

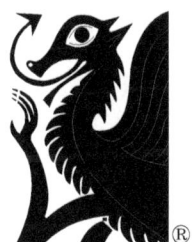

welsh academic press
Cardiff

Published in Wales by Welsh Academic Press, an imprint of

Ashley Drake Publishing Ltd
PO Box 733
Cardiff
CF14 7ZY

www.welsh-academic-press.wales

Hardback edition (2018) 978-1-86057-140-4
Paperback edition (2020) 978-1-86057-144-2
eBook edition (2020) 978-1-86057-150-3

© Ashley Drake Publishing Ltd 2018
Text © Annika Forssén and Gunilla Carlstedt 2018
Translation © Rochelle Wright 2018

The right of Annika Forssén and Gunilla Carlstedt to be identified as the authors of this work has been asserted in accordance with the Copyright Design and Patents Act of 1988.

Every effort has been made to contact copyright holders. However, the publishers will be glad to rectify in future editions any inadvertent omissions brought to their attention.

Ashley Drake Publishing Ltd hereby exclude all liability to the extent permitted by law for any errors or omissions in this book and for any loss, damage or expense (whether direct or indirect) suffered by a third party relying on any information contained in this book.

All rights reserved. No part of this publication may be reproduced, stored in a retrieval system, or transmitted, in any form or by any means without the prior permission of the publishers.

British Library Cataloguing-in-Publication Data.
A CIP catalogue for this book is available from the British Library.

Hardback & paperback editions typeset by Replika Press, India
eBook edition created by Prepress Plus, India (www.prepressplus.in)
Cover design by Welsh Books Council, Aberystwyth, Wales

Contents

Preface   *ix*

Part I: Conversations With Twenty Women   **1**

Introduction   **3**

Selection and interviews   3
From questions to conversations   4
Topic preferences   5
After the interviews   6
Data analysis   7
The twenty women   8

Chapter 1: Growing Up   **12**

Gender and class divisions   12
Brought up to be a woman   13

Chapter 2: Couple Relationships and Social Life   **17**

The single wage-earner family   17
Living alone   18
Becoming a housewife   20
Love – and loneliness   21
Sexuality   22
Married to the husband's job   23
Daily care of husbands   23
Abusive relationships   24
Wife of an alcoholic   25
Divorce   26
A room of one's own   27
Friendships   27
Social relationships   28
Organizational life   29
Political engagement   30
Care of ailing husbands   31
In retrospect   33

Chapter 3: Childbearing — 34

A social issue — 34
Getting pregnant — 36
At the prenatal clinic — 38
Heavy work during pregnancy — 39
Preparing for childbirth — 40
Pain during childbirth — 41
A traumatic experience — 43
Home again — 44
Breastfeeding — 45

Chapter 4: Caring for Children and Other Family Members — 47

Family policy — 47
Motherhood: a mixed blessing — 48
Total responsibility — 48
Availability and vigilance — 49
Around the clock — 50
Training and education — 51
The childcare question — 52
Self-reproach and censure — 53
Father-child relations — 54
A sense of accomplishment — 55
Adult children and grandchildren — 56
Siblings, parents, and other relatives — 57

Chapter 5: Running a Household — 59

Social and political reform — 59
Money and control — 60
The work environment — 61
Cleaning — 63
Laundry — 64
Food preparation — 65
Clothes and other textiles — 66
Guests — 67
In retrospect — 68

Chapter 6: In the Work Force — 70

Women and the labor market — 70
Gender-based salaries — 73

Knowing one's place	75
Sexual harassment	75
Listening and being supportive	76
Time pressure	77
Monotonous and strenuous work	79
On the farm	80
Meaning and pride	81
A room of one's own	82
Work and illness	83
Retirement	84
An adequate pension	85

Chapter 7: Health and Illness — **87**

The welfare state and public health	87
Strong – but fatigued	88
Exhausted due to illness	90
"Aches" – and pain	91
Gynecological "problems"	92
Mental illness	93
Medical treatment	94
Caring for others	95
Maintaining health	96
In old age	97

Chapter 8: Looking Back, and Ahead — **99**

Contentment and sorrow	99
Self-recrimination and shame	100
Reconciliation and hope	101

Part II: Analysis and Discussion — **105**

Introduction — **107**

Chapter 9: Childbearing as Work — **108**

Passive language and active work	108
Prenatal care and women's responsibility	109
The lifelong effects of dismissive treatment	111
Norms and expectations	113

Chapter 10: Unpaid Work — 115

Mothers become home-nurturers — 115
Unseen work — 116
Housework: specialized and strenuous — 117
The husband as a work task — 118
Housework and time — 120
Clock time and process time — 121
Free and restricted time — 122
Older people's time — 123
Unpaid work and health — 123
Summary — 124

Chapter 11: Paid Work — 125

Health benefits — 125
Low status, low pay, and segregation — 127
Bodily contact — 128
Relational work — 129
Sexual harassment — 130
Improved rights – but lack of parity — 131
Sick leave — 133
Work-related injuries — 134
Paid work and time — 135
Career and power within the family — 137
Approaching retirement — 137
Summary — 138

Chapter 12: Illness, Medical Care, and Society — 140

Public healthcare — 140
The medicalization of female biology — 141
Pain and gender — 143
Cardiovascular disease — 144
Mental health issues — 146
Health insurance and women's daily lives — 147
Men's violence against women — 148
Sexualized violence and healthcare — 149
Summary — 151

Chapter 13: Everyday Life and Health — 153

Common symptoms — 153
Fatigue — 153

Compulsive sensitivity	154
Guilt	155
Worry	157
Shame	158
Loneliness	159
Strategies for health	159
A room of one's own	160
Self-determination	161
Making a contribution	162
Culture and creative work	163
Conclusion	**165**
Appendix: Significant Dates in Women's History in Sweden	**168**
References	**173**
English-language publications pertaining to this research project	**185**

Preface

A coffee break conversation at the end of the 1980s was the starting point of our joint research project. In our work as general practitioners we had both noticed that medical knowledge was inadequate or poorly adapted to responding to the health problems many of our female patients described. As a result their symptoms were often dismissed or attributed to psychological disturbances or reproductive biology. By taking another approach – asking women about their life experiences and current situation – we felt we acquired greater insight into their health issues. We became aware that medical science and practice had little knowledge of women's circumstances, their work, paid and unpaid, and the impact of these factors on their health.

Our research got underway a few years later. The goal was to acquire more information about women's work experiences and health. Soon, however, we realized that it was impossible to separate work from other vital matters in women's lives. We also wanted to incorporate insights from other disciplines with medicine. To gather material on women's varied experiences we chose a qualitative research method based on extensive interviews. By selecting older women, we could discern connections and contexts over a long time period. Our findings led to a joint dissertation, published in Swedish as an academic study and then a revised edition published for the more general reader. This book is an English adaptation of these two editions, which has also been revised and updated.

Women in Swedish Society is based on conversations with twenty women, all born in the early 1900s. It begins with a description of our method for collecting and analyzing material and a brief presentation of the women who participated. This is followed by the women's own accounts, organized around various topics. The stories of their lives, from childhood in the 1910s and 1920s until old age in the 1990s, encompass widely divergent personal and work-related experiences; taken together, they provide an overview of Swedish women's history during the twentieth century. We place the women's experiences in the context of typical attitudes and significant events of the time as well as ongoing changes in Swedish society, for instance with regard to legislation, the labor market, and healthcare. In the second part of the book we discuss the women's experiences from the perspective of overarching questions about power, gender, and class, the division of labor between women and men, norms of "femininity," and medical science and practice. Reference is also made to women's circumstances in present-day Sweden and to some degree in other parts of the world.

We ourselves, the authors of the book, have divergent personal and work-related experiences. We grew up in different parts of the country and our class backgrounds are not the same. The work and health histories of our mothers, who were contemporaries of the women in our study, were likewise dissimilar; Annika Forssén's mother was the overburdened wife of a farmer, while Gunilla Carlstedt's was a middle-class housewife in the city. When our research began, Gunilla Carlstedt had five children in young adulthood, whereas Annika Forssén had two small children at home. We thus brought differing perspectives to our joint project. But we also had many points in common: we were both part of a heterosexual couple, and we were both involved in the women's movement that had emerged in the 1960s and '70s with the objective of striving for equality in both the private and the public sphere. Now we also became part of the growing feminist research movement, where the point of departure is placing relations between women and men in focus and taking a stand against the oppression of women wherever it occurs. This approach also incorporated a critical stance toward the perception that (medical) research is objective and unaffected by surrounding social structures. During the course of our work we have become increasingly aware that gender relations must be understood in the context of other social relations and structures. In this book we focus primarily on the connection between gender and class and only touch on questions concerning ethnicity, immigration, sexual orientation and gender identity.

We would like to extend warm and heartfelt thanks to our translator, Rochelle Wright, for her valuable feedback and true engagement with the subject matter. Thanks as well to FORTE (the Swedish Research Council for Health, Working Life and Welfare), which provided funding both for our research and for the translation.

Annika Forssén and
Gunilla Carlstedt
2017

Part I: Conversations with Twenty Women

Introduction

Selection and interviews

The twenty women in our study were born between 1909 and 1929, eighteen of them in Sweden, one in Hungary and one in Finland.[1] All had lived most of their lives in Sweden. At the time of the interviews, 1991-93, they were between 63 and 83 years old. They lived in different parts of the country and were selected stepwise to encompass the widest possible range of work and life experiences, for instance with regard to childhood circumstances, education, occupation, marital status, parenthood, and residence in urban or rural areas.[2] Contact with the women was established through acquaintances, healthcare staff, and organizations of various kinds; they were thus not our own patients. An initial inquiry was made through the contact person and followed up with a letter or telephone call from us, after which the women were given time to think things over. A few women declined to participate because they did not think they had the energy, or were too busy with other matters. Once we had met and interviewed twenty women, no more participants were sought out. We wanted to avoid gathering so much information that it would become unmanageable, and we both wanted to become familiar enough with all the participants that we could recall central portions of their stories without referring to notes.

The conversations took place in the women's homes, in the kitchen or living room. This served to de-emphasize our role as physicians and investigators; we were their guests and needed to adapt to their preferences for how the meeting would proceed. In the context of the home, the women's active, healthy lives and work experiences were more likely to come to mind rather than their illnesses, which would ordinarily have led to contact with physicians. The fact that the women's working lives, not health issues, were the reason for establishing contact in the first place also helped downplay our role as physicians once the interviews began. Each of us met with ten

---

1 In these generations, immigrants to Sweden were few and came primarily from Finland and Eastern Europe.
2 The twenty women who participated are introduced at the end of this chapter.

women, returning to them several times, and consequently we got to know them, and they us. This was essential for them to be comfortable confiding in us about their lives. Between meetings, both participants and interviewers had the opportunity to reflect on and reconsider what had been said. Each conversation lasted between 1.5 and 3 hours and was recorded on tape.

From questions to conversations

The first interview with each woman opened with a question about what had gone through her mind when she was asked to participate in a study focusing on work. After that the interviews were allowed to proceed as relatively unstructured conversations where the women were at liberty to follow their own thoughts and associations. They might then begin talking about matters we did not see as relevant to the topic. Soon, however, we realized that these digressions could lead in new and interesting directions. For instance, it was only after the women insistently returned to the topic of childbearing that the lifelong significance of this experience became clear to us. Allowing the women to tell their stories their own way also helped us avoid some of the terminological confusion that can arise due to differences in cultural background, language use, and so on. The term "sexual harassment," for example, was not very useful. Some did not understand what the expression meant, while others were offended by words suggesting sexual activity. One woman, when asked directly, denied being sexually harassed, but later described this experience spontaneously: "The worst part was going down to the fellows in the cellar. They were incredibly crude, really off-putting. They pinched me and discovered I was ticklish. I was scared to death to go down there."

The unstructured conversations nevertheless made it important not to lose track of matters that we determined were significant before the interviews began or while they were underway. Creating so-called life lines (visual representations with dates and important events written in) together with the women during the interviews was a great aid. These served as a concrete reference point that conversations could evolve from and helped us clarify information about time frames, developments, and connections (Elgqvist-Saltzman 1994: Nilsen 1994). Both during and after the interviews we had additional contact with the women, for instance by letter and phone. The initiative came both from us and from them. They might want to talk about thoughts and memories that had surfaced during the interviews, or about something that had just happened to them. For our part, we felt it was important to know how they were feeling between and after our conversations. Sometimes we could also assist them in their contacts with the healthcare system.

Topic preferences

On a few occasions, interviews left us with the feeling that the women had said "too much." Did they really want to tell us what we had just heard? We never, however, encountered any reactions from the women that confirmed these qualms; instead they showed great trust in us and understood that we were concerned about them as individuals. We realized that our sense of unease arose when we ourselves found something difficult. This experience was reminiscent of our work as physicians, but the situation was different since the responsibility was ours: we had sought out the women, not the other way around. If our conversations brought up matters that were difficult for them, we were accountable, just as we were responsible for the way we reported on our findings.

Some topics turned out to be difficult to talk about, for instance pregnancy prevention, which for some women was beyond the comfort zone. In this instance it was probably a disadvantage to be meeting in their homes rather than a gynecologist's office or medical clinic. From an ethical standpoint it was essential to respect the women's reluctance to speak. No doubt there were also other areas where the women, consciously or unconsciously, were selective about what came out. Presumably they also made some adjustments so as to tell us what they thought we wanted to hear. Difficult periods in life may have been "forgotten" and other matters given a positive twist to enable them to make peace with the way life had turned out. The purpose of biographical studies is seldom to establish a historically accurate "truth" about "how things really were," but rather to find out how a person looking back on life experiences views them from the perspective of the present-day situation (Bjerén 2009: 11). There is also a connection between the way people generate the story of their lives and the way society at large functions. The psychologist Frigga Haug, who has worked extensively with life stories, writes, "In short, we can explore how they inscribe themselves in the existing structures" (Haug 1992: 20). As another psychologist has stressed, relating something has consequences for the way we see ourselves (Magnusson 1997).

Both during and after the interviews it was vital that the women not feel exploited or humiliated. One way of preventing this was to try to end each conversation on a positive note. This was especially important at the final interview. It was essential that the women were left with a sense of strength and dignity after looking back on their lives.

After the interviews

Shortly after each interview, we listened to the tape together and wrote up a detailed summary. The new insights this gave us affected subsequent conversations with the same woman, and with others. Listening together also allowed us to share our sense of how the interview had gone, to comment on each other's impression of what the women had said and to discuss what we at that stage considered important or relevant to the topic. We could uncover each other's blind spots, for instance things we had not "heard" or had let pass without follow-up questions, or perhaps had misunderstood. In this connection it was beneficial that our own experiences, in childhood and later in life, differed significantly. It was also a pleasure to exchange thoughts and conjectures.

Both of us worked with the narratives of all twenty women. Although we had each met only half of them in person, over time we became so familiar with their stories that toward the end of the analytical process we both felt we knew them all. Tapes and transcriptions also made it possible to verify that we had not distorted the women's statements or drawn conclusions that could not be supported.

The interviews were transcribed literally. As work proceeded, we had become increasingly aware that tape recordings could not convey the conversations in full. Transcriptions led to a further reduction or loss of relevant information. For that reason it was important to listen to the tapes, not only to hear the women's voices but also to recall, relive, and tell each other about facial expressions and body language that accompanied their stories. This helped us assess the significance of what had just been said. When the women are quoted in the book we have occasionally made minor adjustments to clarify what they meant. Spoken language can often seem dull in print, where inflection is lacking. Quotations can thus come across as naïve or stripped down. Our goal was both to make them read smoothly and to do the women justice (compare Kvale 1996/2009: 177-83). Our editing consisted of eliminating repetitions or phrases and digressions that were difficult to follow. Quotations from the same woman were sometimes merged when they addressed the same topic and gave a more nuanced picture when taken together.

Initially we intended that the women read part or all of the transcripts from their own interviews, but none of them wished to. Some did, however, request copies of the relevant tape recordings.

Data analysis

The analysis of the women's stories began at the same moment as the interviews: our interpretation of the women's stories, responses, and reactions determined the way conversations proceeded. New, unanticipated questions and follow-up questions came up as well. When we listened to the tapes and wrote and read through the summaries we identified additional subjects to be investigated. Alongside this we familiarized ourselves with relevant theoretical approaches and research results within medicine and other fields, primarily feminist/women's studies. In this manner theory and empirical data enriched and reinforced each other.

We began a systematic process of analysis by reading through two interviews apiece, choosing women who were as different from each other as possible. The first reading was to identify areas and themes in the interviews, initially divided into "work", defined broadly, and "health or ill health." Through these women's stories we could identify, at an early stage, several themes under "work", such as household work, relational work, childbearing, and so on. Concerning health issues, we decided to use the broad, non-specific themes of "wellbeing" and "suffering". These themes were used and new themes identified as we went through the remaining interviews. For example, themes such as "significant conditions for health/ill health" and "encountering healthcare" were added.

Statements that fit into the various themes were highlighted and assigned a tag in the margin of the transcript. We then wrote out central portions of the statements we had marked – referred to in the literature as condensed "meaning units" – in the form of word-for-word quotations ranging from a few words to one or two sentences. This was done by hand, on slips of paper, while at the same time placing these under the relevant heading (coding). The women's pseudonymous names, the interview number and page number were recorded on the slips of paper so the quotations could easily be found in the original text. The stacks of paper of various heights that resulted from this "handiwork" gave us a visual image of the content of the stories. We gained a first impression of how the individual women had apportioned their time and their involvement in relationships and various kinds of work and to what degree wellbeing and/or suffering played a role in their lives. The quotations were then entered on the computer, organized according to themes, but still tied to particular women. After this we reorganized the entire material so that quotations from all twenty women were collected under these rubrics. The next step was to create subtitles: under "work", for instance, categories included responsibility, heavy work, and time constraints. The entire analysis process was inspired by Tesch's (1990) and Giorgi's (1985) methods for qualitative analysis. We continued by writing short summaries of the content of the various subthemes, giving them new descriptive titles and sometimes creating new concepts to express what they encompassed. We also linked findings within themes and subthemes to each other, for example connecting "childbearing" to "encountering healthcare."

Rather than following the life lines of individual women, we now had a "cross-section"[3] of the material, allowing us to see the variety in the women's work assignments and experiences, and similarities as well as differences among them. This step put the quotations at an even greater remove from their original context, so it was essential that both of us were very familiar with all the women. To support the analysis and to see the connections in every woman's life, we summarized each individual account and wrote it out as a life story. The rubrics were essentially the same as in the "cross-sectional analysis" but the chronology was adjusted to fit the individual life stories. The life lines we had created with the women were a big help in this. One of our articles explicitly combines these two analytical methods (Forssén, Carlstedt and Mörtberg 2005). Another tells an individual woman's story against the background of contemporary historical events (Carlstedt 2009).

The twenty women

The women's names are pseudonymous

Anna, b. 1913. Grew up in foster home in the country. No chance to continue education past primary school. Married into farm family with country store. Four children. Wide scope of strenuous work. Always many people on the farm. Active in several organizations. Cared for mother-in-law suffering from senile dementia. Widow. Early heart attack, difficult-to-treat angina, chronic back problems. Disability pension at age 54. Helped children and grandchildren. Cherished her happy memories.

Blenda, b. 1910. Grew up on farm on an island. In charge of farm and younger siblings in early adulthood. Later lived in large city. Married, one child; chose to divorce early. Remarried later in life. Worked as a maid, kitchen assistant, and homecare provider. Retired at 65. Widow. Survived cancer and a heart attack. Close contact with daughter and grandchildren. Cultural interests enriched her life.

---

3 The term "cross-sectional" has a different meaning in quantitative research.

Britt-Marie, b. 1929. Grew up in middle-class family in medium-sized town. Graduated from secondary school. Single, no children. Entire working life at same government agency. Down-graded in reorganization. Cared for ailing father, no close relatives after his death. Periods of depression, arthritis of the hip and mild diabetes. Disability pension at age 62. Strong interest in music and art.

Edit, b. 1914. Grew up on family farm. Lived in large city after marriage. Two children. Worked in husband's grocery shop. Enjoyed housework and work in the shop. Continued working for pay until age 72. Widow. Partially paralyzed after stroke, putting effort into rehabilitation. Significant contact with children, grandchildren, extended family, friends. Keenly interested in people.

Elina, b. 1922. Grew up on a farm in Finland. Lost several family members during the war, serious hip injury at age 14 working in the forest. Mourned lack of education. Came to Sweden shortly after the war; ongoing contact with relatives in Finland. Difficult marriage to Swedish factory worker from the Finnish-speaking minority. Repeated miscarriages. Gave birth to two children, one deceased at birth. Cleaner and daycare teacher, enjoyed her work. Chronic hip problems, heart attack. Disability pension at age 56. Active in clubs and organizations. Close contact with daughter and grandchildren. Enjoyed banter and joking.

Elna, b. 1919. Small-town upbringing. Married to military officer, divorced early. Three children, one put up for adoption. Worked as hairdresser, at odd jobs, and in factories. Proud of her work life. Cared for relatives and other people's children. Rheumatoid arthritis, surgery for kidney cancer, impaired vision. Disability pension at age 57. Provided extensive help to children and grandchildren. Always interested in expanding her horizons.

Estrid, b. 1909. Parents indentured agricultural laborers. Worked outside the home from an early age. Later city dweller, married to unskilled laborer. Five children, one killed in accident as a teenager. Worked in restaurants, in homes, cleaning up building sites. Pension at age 63. Cared for ailing husband. Widow. Heart problems, diabetes, arthritis – but felt healthy. Close contact with children and grandchildren.

Frida, b. 1924. Grew up in lower middle-class home, married to civil servant. No children. Nurse. Frequently ill, many abdominal operations. Periods of depression. Alongside job, cared for ailing husband and mother. Disability pension at age 59. Kept up her strength through exercise classes and dance. Loved jazz.

Gertrud, b. 1924. Grew up on family farm. Married to civil servant, two children. Strove for equality in her marriage. Nurse, healthcare teacher. Salaried work important, but quit at age 63 due to dissatisfaction. Hearing loss beginning around age 40. Active in clubs and organizations. Close contact with children and grandchildren, pleased about their progress toward gender equality.

Greta, b. 1926. Grew up on family farm. Midwife. Married to minister, many duties related to his position. Psychologically abusive husband. Four children and several foster children. Profession and charitable work important. High blood pressure, defective heart valve, heart attack. Pension at 64. Separated from husband. Close contact with children and grandchildren. Choral singing and playing the piano lifted her spirits.

Irina, b. 1922. Middle-class upbringing in Hungary. Married during wartime, husband civil engineer. Three children. Home destroyed during the war. Fled to Sweden under dangerous circumstances in the 1950s. A housewife by choice. Churchwarden for a few years before retirement. Close contact with children and grandchildren. Healthy and content.

Karin, b. 1912. Grew up in middle-class family. Trained as dental hygienist, quit after marriage. Many duties connected with husband's job as school administrator. Two children. Enjoyed work in the home and for husband and children. Widow. Vision, hearing, and joint problems. No grandchildren. Contact with many friends. On the go.

Klary, b. 1913. Grew up in poverty in large city. Married, chose not to have children. Both husband and wife factory workers. Quit at age 63 due to fatigue. Cared for older, ailing husband. Widow. No close relatives. Back pain, mild diabetes. Kept her spirits up.

Linnea, b. 1926. Grew up in upper middle-class family. Physician, married to a physician. Felt isolated due to lack of respect from husband. Four children, one psychologically handicapped. At home with children for fifteen years against her will. Divorced. Burned out professionally. Suffered heart attack. Retired at 65. Helped children and grandchildren. Fulfilling many dreams in old age.

Malin, b. 1909. Middle-class upbringing in large city. Secretarial school, married to civil servant. Three children, one deceased in adulthood. Always worked outside the home, supported family. Enjoyed her job as executive secretary; pension at 65. Husband periodically depressed and unemployed. Widow. Basically healthy. Did not want to be a burden to her children. Active and satisfied with her life.

Marta, b. 1910. Grew up on family farm. Wanted an education. Became a teacher, then an artist. In committed relationship, but choose not to cohabit. No children. Cared for nieces and nephews. Many friends and close contact with younger relatives. Nearly blind but still active professionally at age 83. Created "survival pictures."

Sara, b. 1920. Upper middle-class upbringing in large city.

Secondary school teacher, married to colleague. Mourned lack of equality in marriage. Two children. Very happy in her profession, retired reluctantly at 64. Ailing husband needed care in old age. Joint pain, slight angina. Close contact with children and grandchildren. Organizational involvement. Valued women friends and supported women's rights.

Signe, b. 1920. Grew up in extreme poverty. Married at seventeen. Lived on isolated island without modern conveniences. Ten children, one deceased in adulthood. Widowed when children were still young. Economic privation, no help from social welfare agencies. Angina and defective heart valve, back pain. Active in clubs and organizations. Helped children and grandchildren. Felt she had made a contribution.

Valborg, b. 1912. Grew up in poverty on small farm. Worked in agriculture. Married, later moved to city. Cleaner. Husband an alcoholic, difficult daily life. Three children, one deceased at birth. Disability pension at age 63. Worn out from taking care of verbally abusive, ailing husband in old age. Felt unappreciated. Chronic urinary tract problems, back and neck pain. Helped children and grandchildren, pleased that they helped her in return.

Vera, b. 1924. Grew up on small farm. Engineer. Lived alone, no children. Chose career rather than family. Difficulties as a woman in male-dominated profession. Actively involved in organizations and politics. Arthritis of the knee, Stein-Leventhal's syndome (endochrinological disease). Retired reluctantly at 64 due to diminished job satisfaction, but remained proud of her competence.

1

Growing Up

Gender and class divisions

In the 1910s and 1920s, when the women we interviewed were growing up, Sweden remained an impoverished country. Industrialization was gaining ground, but a significant portion of the population found its livelihood in the agricultural sector and in forestry. Most people, both in rural areas and in cities, lived in crowded conditions and without access to modern amenities such as indoor plumbing. Poor health was also more widespread than it is today; substandard, unhygienic housing and malnutrition contributed to the spread of disease. Particularly during World War I (1914-18), food supplies were inadequate in many areas.[4] Infectious diseases such as tuberculosis, pneumonia, measles and diphtheria claimed many lives, as did the 1918 influenza pandemic referred to as the Spanish flu.

Society was structured around a strict division of labor between men and women, according to which women were responsible for caregiving and running the household while men were expected to be the primary breadwinners. Medical science offered biological arguments against women working in the public sector, claiming they were unsuitable for such employment due to lower intellectual and reasoning skills and furthermore would compromise their reproductive capabilities. These limitations, however, applied primarily to women from the middle and upper classes; on farms and in factories, women's work outside the home was often a necessity, both to support individual families and for society at large to function. Compared to men, women of all social classes had limited political, economic and legal rights.

Not all women accepted these unequal conditions. Beginning in the nineteenth century, radical political groups and various women's

---

4 Sweden was not a combatant, but was largely cut off from the rest of the world.

organizations had championed a more independent role and expanded opportunities for women, asserting that they should have the same degree of control over their lives as men did. An important milestone on the road toward self-determination came in 1921, when after a long struggle women won the right to vote in political elections. Also in that year, married women gained rights of majority (which unmarried women had possessed since 1858) and were authorized to manage their own money.

At the beginning of the previous century women received very little information about their bodily functions. Contributing factors were inadequate healthcare, lack of resources, and prevailing social attitudes. In part because of this ignorance, sexual activity, both within and outside marriage, and childbearing gave rise to major health risks, including sexually transmitted diseases, other infections, and hemorrhaging. Women were also vulnerable because it was illegal in Sweden to provide information about or sell contraceptives, a ban put into effect in 1910, prompted by moral fervor and concerns about diminishing birthrates (it was lifted in 1938). The number of unplanned pregnancies as well as the spread of venereal disease could have been significantly reduced if contraceptives and information about pregnancy prevention had been available.

Many women facing unplanned pregnancies tried to resolve the situation by having abortions. Since this procedure was also illegal, it often took place under unhygienic conditions and the mortality rate was high, especially for women in lower socio-economic groups; those who survived were often left sterile. If the story got out, those who had undergone or sought out abortions could be sentenced to prison. Women's right to determine over their own bodies with regard to sexuality and childbearing, and thus avoid many of the related hazards, was not achieved until much later in the twentieth century (see Chapter 3, Childbearing). Legislation addressing sexual abuse and men's violence against women was likewise a later development (see Chapter 12).

Brought up to be a woman

Many of the women in our study came from families with limited economic resources. Schooling was brief and they were expected to join the adult female work force as children. Estrid, who grew up among indentured farm laborers, described having to pitch in and help her mother clean houses at the age of twelve. In farm families it was taken for granted that girls would help their mothers with cooking, baking, dishwashing and tidying. "Goodness, how we worked!" exclaimed Blenda, whose family owned a farm on an island in the Baltic. "There was no end to the things you needed to learn. When I was ten I made two batches of bread, one white, the other rye. My hands knew how much flour to use." Several women remembered the sense of connection that working with their mothers had provided. Others thought it was unfair that their brothers were spared household work and consequently had more time for rest and play. Most women had memories of boys being considered "important" and girls having to wait on their brothers. "We had to iron our brothers' suits," Elna recalled.

Some of the women had lost their mothers early in life. At nine, when her mother died, Linnea felt that the only person who had noticed and listened to her was gone. Rather than receiving comfort and support, she felt pressured to assume her mother's role as listener. "You're brought up to be considerate of everyone, to be there for everyone," she said. Other girls had to take over the workload of deceased or sickly mothers. Elina remembered her father's words when her mother became bedridden and she had to drop out of school: "You can't go to school – who would take care of the animals?" Neither did Anna get the education she had hoped for. After her mother died when she was twelve, she was placed in a foster home. Aware of her outsider status, she never dared ask her foster parents whether she could continue after the obligatory six years of primary school, nor did anyone ask what she preferred.

Blenda attended a rural school of household management, but after her parents died she was forced to cut short her education to take care of younger siblings and the family farm. Marta, who lost her mother when she was sixteen, was likewise expected to take on responsibility for a large rural household. She nevertheless felt a strong desire to study and get out in the world and was not willing to accept the fate of staying at home to run the farm. To get her way she deliberately took drastic action: "I let a skillet of pork and peas burn so badly that smoke filled the house. After that my father decided I was hopeless at household tasks and let me enroll at a folk high school."

Even in families that were well off, it was by no means self-evident that girls would continue their education. When Malin, who grew up in a middle-class family, was encouraged by a teacher to ask her father if she could attend secondary school, his response was a flat-out no because he did not think she had a convincing argument for just what use that would be.[5] Later on Malin attended secretarial school, a

---

5 This was at the time when Swedish girls were admitted to public secondary schools (1927). Previously, those who wished to pursue a higher education attended private girls' schools. However, women were granted the right to earn a university degree as early as 1873, though the fields of law and theology remained closed to them.

common career path for women of her social class. Because there were servants in her home, she was among those who learned very little about housekeeping while she was young. This was also the case with girls whose families encouraged their educational goals from the beginning; domestic skills were seen as unnecessary and as taking too much time away from studying. Later in life, when these women married and had families of their own, they were nevertheless expected to know how to take care of their homes, husbands and children.

Some women who had grown up in poverty had mothers who very actively supported their desire for an education; they wanted their daughters to have the opportunity for a better life than they themselves had had. Even so, it was not always possible for girls to get the education and training that most appealed to them. Though Frida wanted to be a teacher, her mother borrowed money so she could train as a nurse; healthcare offered more opportunities for temporary positions that could support her during her studies. That Vera would continue in school was taken for granted. She dreamed of studying literature, but the family's limited economic resources could only accommodate training that would lead to a job. Vera was one of two girls attending a technical secondary school, where she studied engineering. Elna had been encouraged by her mother to get an education so she "wouldn't be dependent on a man." She became a hairdresser. The girls' prospects for continuing their education and choosing a profession were thus determined by their sex, but also by finances, social class, and place of residence.

Since girls were often ill-informed about female physiology, many were taken aback by the physical changes associated with puberty. This ignorance was the same in all social classes. Klary, who grew up in urban poverty, related, "When I got my first period around age thirteen, I had no idea what it was, and I didn't dare ask, either. I don't know what I did." Blenda, from a rural background, was equally unprepared. After receiving an explanation, she remembered sobbing and screaming that she didn't want to be a girl. Sara, from an intellectual, urban, middle-class family, was likewise completely ignorant of how her body worked.

The silence, and even prejudice, that surrounded them gave many girls a negative image of their own bodies and their own sex. Sexual feelings were considered off limits and shameful. Linnea, the future physician, recalled a book her older brother had shown her: "It said that a woman shouldn't pump the pedals of her sewing machine when she was having her period because this might cause sexual arousal." The unwritten rules of sexual conduct were also extremely strict. "The degree of fear associated with sex was unbelievable," said Blenda. The anxiety the girls sensed from adults, particularly their mothers, concerned the risk of pregnancy. Blenda recalled one occasion when she was punished for attending a dancing party – she was too young, her mother thought – while a younger brother who had been at the same gathering was not reprimanded. Only later in life did Blenda realize that her mother's overreaction was triggered by her awareness of the shame and social stigma experienced by unwed mothers; she knew from personal experience, since she herself had been a "bastard" – a word used well into the twentieth century to designate children born out of wedlock.

Women born early in the previous century thus faced many constraints and limitations, including economic privation, legal barriers, gender-based social attitudes, and the expectations and demands of family. Negotiating these restrictions to self-determination and finding satisfaction and fulfillment in life was a challenge that women met in many different ways and with varying degrees of success.

2

Couple Relationships and Social Life

The single wage-earner family

The women in this study reached adulthood during the 1930s and '40s, a period noted for social reforms in which the goal was to increase the country's overall standard of living. The Social Democrats' ascent to political power in 1932 is generally seen as the first step toward the establishment of a People's Home. The latter was Prime Minister Per Albin Hansson's term for an equal society, without privileged or neglected groups and with systems of security embracing everyone, irrespective of social class.[6]

Marriage between a man and a woman was considered one of the essential foundations upon which society was built. The political ideal of the husband as sole wage earner, which previously had applied to the bourgeoisie, now began to include working-class families. The message to *all* women was that their primary place was in the home, with the mission of running the household and caring for husband and children. Proposals that women should receive obligatory instruction in household management were taken up periodically, with particular emphasis on the importance of this initiative for working-class women. The economic crisis that struck the entire western world during the 1930s, bringing large-scale unemployment, contributed to strengthening the ideal of the stay-at-home wife, since the argument was that women should not take jobs away from men. Another problem was the diminishing birthrate, which during the mid-1930s fell to the lowest levels of the century. This circumstance was ascribed to economic conditions: young people simply could not afford to start a family. Various welfare reforms, such as housing allowances, were designed to promote marriage and increase childbearing.

---

6 What this entailed for the everyday lives of women is described in Chapter 5, Running a Household.

For unattached women, the situation remained difficult, especially for those with children, since they were excluded from the family model promoted by the political power structure. In all occupations, women earned less than men; in typically female occupations wages were so low that a single woman could scarcely support herself or afford housing. In other words, the focus on family during this period did not encompass what was best for *all* children and adults, but rather what was best for the intact heterosexual family.

Simultaneously the struggle continued to ensure that women and men, regardless of marital status, would have the same prospects and choices in life. In this regard Gunnar and Alva Myrdal played a central role. In their book, *Crisis in the Population Question* (Myrdal and Myrdal 1934) the couple underscored the need for social reform that would make it easier for women to pursue a career as well as give birth to and rear children. In a later book, *Woman, Family and Society*, Alva Myrdal and other radical women expanded further on these ideas. Topics addressed included women's low wages, opportunities for women to gain political influence, marriage on equal terms and ways of combining motherhood and gainful employment (Myrdal et al. 1938).

Same-sex relationships remained a concealed phenomenon in Swedish society until much later in the century. Until 1944 homosexuality was a crime; thereafter, until 1979, it was considered a disease. That certain historically documented close and co-habiting friendships between women were love relationships has only recently been openly acknowledged.[7]

Living alone

Despite the dominant family model of the period, some of the women interviewed had ruled out marriage from the start. The burden of housekeeping and caregiving that they would be expected to take on if they "started a family" was not what they wanted or felt they could handle, especially with regard to waiting on a husband.

Marta, who initially became a teacher and later a professional artist, explained that for many years she refrained from long-term relationships and the possibility of children so she would be free

---

7 Among the most prominent Swedish women involved in such relationships were Selma Lagerlöf (1858-1940), writer and Nobel Prize winner; Karin Boye (1900-1941), writer; and Barbro Alving – "Bang" – (1909-1987), journalist and writer.

to work. "I didn't dare get married; I felt I had to choose." Later in life she did have an ongoing relationship with a man that provided emotional and intellectual companionship, but she still insisted on living alone despite the man's wish to cohabit. "I think it's quite necessary for a woman to have time for herself," she said. "I would never have been able to work the way I did if we had lived together." Vera, the engineer, also spoke of having to make a choice. "If I had married, I would have ended up in a boring job or been forced to start over," she said, though she might have been willing to make this sacrifice if she had found someone who met her requirements, a man who was "reasonably intellectual," as she put it. Friends thought she was "too picky," but she herself felt that women often fared badly in marriage and family life, especially if they had little in common with their husbands. That was not what she wanted.

Blenda had married, but got a divorce as soon as she became aware that her husband was a chronic alcoholic. She was pregnant and had nowhere to live; divorce was uncommon and considered shameful. Even so, she chose to strike out on her own and lived alone with her child for many years. "I didn't trust men," she said. Elna had realized on her wedding day that the marriage probably would not last. She had never been especially interested in "finding a man," but had become pregnant. "If it had happened today, I would never have gotten married. In those days you had to," she said. Later, when her husband asked for a divorce, she was nevertheless ashamed to be the only one she knew who "couldn't make a go of it." Over time she felt fine about the divorce and lived alone for the rest of her life. She wanted to "read in the evening, go to the movies, get together with friends, not be stuck taking care of a man."

Britt-Marie likewise chose not to get married, but for a different reason: she saw it as a "terrible responsibility" she was not up to. "A man won't make a commitment to someone who doesn't wait on him," she said, thus demonstrating that she had internalized the then-dominant perception of a woman's role in marriage. She did have two long-term relationships with men, one of them a military officer, but could never bring herself to become his wife because she did not feel up to assuming the hostess duties this role would require.

Being single was nonetheless problematic for women, since it had a negative effect on social position. "The status of unmarried women is lower than for married women," stated Vera. She and several others also experienced difficulties finding decent housing. "If you were single, all you could get was a little room they called 'old maids' digs'," Vera continued. The teachers' quarters where Marta was put up had no running water or toilet and was heated by a wood-burning stove.

When she requested improvements she was told, "If you get married, Missy, things will work out." A male colleague with a stay-at-home wife, on the other hand, was assumed to need modern facilities.

Becoming a housewife

Remaining unmarried was nevertheless an uncommon choice for women of this generation, and women in the study generally regarded marriage to a man as an explicit goal in life. Physical attraction and falling in love were motivating factors, but marriage also represented economic security and might be the only possibility of establishing a "real home." Irina, who grew up in Hungary, related that occupational training and working outside the home were considered out of the question. Getting married thus became "a kind of life insurance," as she put it. For a couple of women, the desire to have a home of their own was so powerful that they married men they knew they did not love. Such was the choice for Valborg, working as a live-in farm laborer, still hoping marriage would bring a better life, but in vain.

One question that became relevant soon after marriage was whether the women would continue working outside the home. When Estrid's husband did not want her to work, she saw this as proof of his love as well as a chance to escape her poorly-paid, exhausting job for a while. One assumption of the arrangement was that she would take care of her husband in the way he expected. Karin, who had trained to be a dental hygienist, also let her husband decide that she would work only within the home. For both these women, their husbands' preference for a stay-at-home wife was in keeping with their own wishes.

Not so for the physician Linnea, who remained at home for many years against her will. One of her children was handicapped and she felt she had no choice, since neither her husband nor social services offered any help. Most of the other women who had trained for a profession nevertheless remained in the work force, though their common experience was that they also bore primary responsibility for home and children. Those who continued did not, however, always encounter encouragement and support from their husbands. When Sara, who taught science in secondary school, started working on a doctorate in biology, her husband's dismissive comments about her competence were one reason she did not continue.

Love – and loneliness

When the women talked about their married lives, some focused primarily on friendship and love. "I really did love him, and he loved me. We were very close," said Klary. She recalled happy times with her husband when they were home alone. "He loved dancing, so we rolled up the rug and danced." Others described a sense of connection, of support and assistance when the workload was heavy or when they were ill. "He wanted me to have help if I needed it – he was very tender-hearted," said Edit, a mother of two and married to a greengrocer. Signe, who had ten children, also mentioned her husband's explicit support. "He often said, 'You can clean the house when the kids are grown up – don't worry about that now.'" Her husband's concern for the children was an important component of her marital experience. Anna, married to a farmer, described a silent understanding that had evolved between husband and wife over the years. "It was as though we could read each other's thoughts."

Others' experience was that their husbands claimed center stage and demanded to be waited on from the very beginning. Greta, the midwife, described newlywed life as "waking up from a blue-eyed dream." She had viewed her husband, who was in divinity school, as "a kind, considerate person," but now he began organizing drinking parties in their one-room apartment. She herself was pregnant and also supporting the family. "I needed my sleep, but there wasn't much chance of that." In order to get through it, she had reminded herself, "I'll just have to get used to it – this is my new life."

Several women described loneliness and alienation. "The years I was married I didn't feel so great, because I was always alone," said Elna. Elina, who emigrated from Finland and married a Swedish man, expressed her disappointment with these words: "I've never really been able to talk to him. I guess being alone is just the way it is." Linnea, the physician, had met her husband in medical school, but discovered immediately after their marriage that he expected her to be at his beck and call. "That sense of teamwork was completely gone. Everything was extremely pleasant and we had a good life – as long as I kept myself in check and didn't make demands." Loneliness in the marriage would subsequently trouble her for years. "Among my colleagues I was very highly regarded, but in my private life I counted for nothing." For a long time she expected her husband to notice and try to modify the imbalance in circumstances and decision-making power that had arisen between them. Her reluctance to insist that he take on a larger share of the housework and caregiving responsibilities had eventually led, she believed, to the periods of depression she suffered. Still other women cited their dislike of "shouting and screaming" as a reason they had avoided making demands. Many years later the memories were still painful. "I don't like talking about it – it hurts so much inside," said Sara, placing her hand over her heart. At the same time she was upset with herself for having been so "bad about expressing what I wanted."

Sexuality

Many of the women were not accustomed to talking about sexuality, a topic that in the mid-twentieth century was more taboo than it is today. Some implied that their sexual experiences had been mutually satisfying. "Especially when we were young, it was good," said Klary. The sexual connection could nevertheless vary over time, in significance as well as intensity. Gertrud described it this way: "You wanted to be together that way, too, but over the years it has shifted, gone up and down. Sometimes you were too tired, didn't always feel in the mood. But we're a lot alike, my husband and me. He hasn't been insistent, and besides, he's so sensitive that if things weren't good between us, he wasn't interested, either." She added, "But maybe he was disappointed sometimes – being a wife or a lover was never my first priority." Linnea described a sexual attraction that initially was strong but soon faded. It was primarily her husband who lost interest, which caused her great distress and disappointment.

A number of women described agreeing to have sex because their husbands demanded it and to avoid a fight. Valborg's husband had told her that sex was "expected," something she had to go along with whether or not it gave her pleasure. Even Klary, who had been "eager for sex" when she was young, admitted that later in life it was mostly unpleasant and she had gone along with it "to keep the peace at home."

The minister's wife Greta, who in a previous relationship had experienced sex as "great," was completely unprepared for the problems that developed in her marriage. Her husband was often impotent, a condition she had previously never even heard of. Time after time she had felt obligated to "help" him without deriving any pleasure from this herself. "I'm sure I'll get it up next time," was her husband's comment after each failed attempt. "The odd thing was," she continued, "that he could satisfy himself, though he didn't think this was natural. But it was natural for me to do what he wanted." Eventually she realized she had a right to say no, but had believed the relationship would suffer if she did.

Married to the husband's job

Edit was among the women who assumed part of the workload connected to her husband's job as soon as she was married. He was a grocer, and to her, working alongside him was both enjoyable and a given. For many years they ran the shop together. Anna, the farmer's wife, who took on responsibility for a large household, barn animals, and a country store from the day she wed, also felt a bond with her husband through work.

After her husband was ordained, the midwife Greta was thrown into a daily routine that encompassed many tasks connected with his work. These included church coffees, meetings with confirmation classes, funerals and other church events. She was also expected to be active in various charity organizations, and the minister's home was supposed to be open to visitors at all times, including for meals and overnight stays. As the minister's wife, she was always the hostess, and she had no household help. On Sundays her husband wanted her to be at services: "So I set the table and got everything ready, put the coffee pot on low, and then we left for church. I had all the children with me. When we got home the coffee was ready. Then I could stand there receiving guests. Afterwards I did the dishes and vacuumed so things would be in order if new visitors turned up." She scarcely received any recognition for her contribution. She remembered the speeches when her husband retired. Neither her husband nor members of the congregation mentioned all the years she had worked at her husband's side. "I felt as if I were sinking through the floor. I thought, what about me? It seemed to me that I'd truly worked my fingers to the bone." A few weeks later Greta had her first heart attack.

Karin was a stay-at-home wife when her husband became principal of a secondary school. For Karin this meant organizing large dinner parties and setting up guest rooms for overnight visitors. Unlike the minister's wife, who had to manage with extremely limited financial resources, Karin could employ hired help for cooking, serving, and cleaning, and moreover her husband noticed and appreciated what she did. Even so, he never bought the car she longed for. A car would have made it easier for her to shop, but he felt it was unnecessary and she did not press him: "He would give me the moon and the stars if I asked, but I didn't want to nag."

Daily care of husbands

While growing up, most of the women had been taught that one anticipated task in life would be to wait on their husbands. This made some of them feel needed, even indispensable, and the care they voluntarily gave their husbands created a bond – if it was acknowledged and appreciated. Even in marriages where both husband and wife were employed outside the home, some women had viewed it as natural that they personally would wait on their husbands. Klary, who for most of her life worked at the same factory as her husband, described going to and from work together, but at home in the evening she was the one who fixed dinner while he lay down on the sofa with the newspaper. "That's how people thought things should be," she said.

A number of women stated that their responsibilities had increased over the years as their husbands became more dependent on their services. Some used phrases such as "being like a mother" or "he was like a child" when describing this development. Much of this daily concern had to do with health issues. It was the women who facilitated contact with healthcare providers, even if their husbands were not seriously ill. Women also saw to it that their husbands ate nutritious food and tried to change their eating habits to promote health. Often they were the ones who made accommodations. "I thought we should meet halfway," said Elina, "but he wanted to eat the food he was used to." Several women also mentioned that when they were away and the men had to fend for themselves, they were utterly inept in the kitchen. "Coffee, maybe he could boil that. I had cooked and put things in the freezer but it didn't help. He couldn't manage on his own at all," Blenda, remarried in her 50s, recalled.

Many women also described providing encouragement and a listening ear. They had learned how to read their husbands' mood changes and cope with temper flare-ups while sparing them their own troubles. "I've backed him up in every way, let him devote himself to his work," said Greta, the minister's wife. Only later in life did certain women question the accommodations they made and the service role they provided to satisfy their husbands' demands or creature comforts. Though Linnea was aware early on of an imbalance in caretaking roles, it still took many years before she fully realized how much she had contributed to making her husband's everyday life run smoothly. Klary thought her husband had been "spoiled."

Abusive relationships

Several women described overtly controlling behavior on the part of their husbands. Elina had to deal with her husband's hot temper on a daily basis. Tact and restraint helped her avoid conflict: "You have to be careful what you talk about, not tease – that makes him furious." Greta felt that for a long time she let her husband dominate her, blaming this on her low self-esteem. He was "like a master" who wanted control over everything she did and insisted she follow the rules he set up. "If I wanted to play the piano, I had to see to it that the countertop was completely clean first, and while I was playing he just stood there, staring." Having "nerves of steel" was necessary to get through the daily routines, she felt. "Sometimes I didn't know from one second to the next how I'd get through the next second. I was so distraught that I sometimes went out in a snowstorm. I couldn't stand listening to him any more." But it was not always that way. "There were calm periods, too – he was nice sometimes," she said. "If he'd made me really miserable, things would be fine for a while." The fact that her husband retained sole control of family finances also made her feel she had been declared incompetent. Since he was stingy, it was extremely difficult for her to cover household expenses. "No one knew how little money I had," she related. When her husband suffered periods of depression he became even more domineering, while she in turn became more accommodating for fear of making the illness worse or "causing a relapse." For her own peace of mind she learned to take advantage of moments of freedom. "Things were best for me when he was out of the house because then I could do more or less what I pleased," she commented. Eventually she began protesting more openly against his controlling behavior. Looking back, she was convinced she had been psychologically abused.

None of the women who felt oppressed in their marriages told anyone, not even their closest women friends. "You were completely alone – it was impossible to talk about it," said Elina. As a reason for their silence, they cited not wanting to "expose" their husbands, children, or themselves. They also described feeling a personal responsibility for the way their marriages had evolved. This made them unsure of themselves: if they did tell someone, would they be met with understanding or accusations?

Wife of an alcoholic

A couple of the women had lived with men who abused alcohol. Valborg stayed in a marriage in which her husband's alcoholism and utter lack of responsibility affected every aspect of her life. She lost control and never knew what might happen. "Never being able to rely on him, that was the worst of it." Was he drunk or not? Would he decide to take the car out for a spin? Start a fire by smoking in bed? Disturb the neighbors? That he often drank up the money needed to run the household made daily life even more difficult for the family. Their friendships and social life were also constrained. Sometimes she had to turn away visitors, even children and grandchildren, because she did not know what shape her husband would be in. At the same time her husband's abuse made her feel guilty and accountable. She felt she had "done him an injustice" since she never could bring herself to love him.

For Estrid, the difficulties connected with her husband's abuse were not as major, as long as she made certain accommodations. "He drank some, quite a lot sometimes, came home and picked a fight," she related. Since she loved her husband and felt loved by him, she chose not to get upset every time this happened. If she wanted to live with him, she would have to put up with sporadic drinking bouts and fights.

Divorce

As previously described, Marta and Vera established their own spheres in life by never marrying, while Blenda and Elna did so by divorcing early on. Linnea, the physician, eventually chose divorce as well. After leaving her husband she felt a sense of relief about "being spared the irritation of constantly seeing how things could be but never were," but the divorce was also painful, since she continued to grieve about a marriage where she had felt unnoticed and unloved. As a divorcée she could nevertheless seek out experiences she had longed for. "I had a fellow for a few years," she related, "since I wanted some more sex in my life and he was good at that." But when he began "settling in on my sofa" she broke off the relationship. She wanted to be free.

For others, things never got past the thinking stage. "I'm not sure there's much point getting divorced now," said Elina. At the time of the interview she was ill and felt her husband provided some support in spite of everything. "But I wonder sometimes," she continued. "Is this really what married life should be like?" It was hard to stop thinking about "a little place of my own." Valborg, the alcoholic's wife, had likewise considered divorce. "But there were the kids," she said. "How would they have felt if they'd seen him wandering around town like a tramp?" At one point she had contacted an attorney, but that was as far as it went. The minister's wife Greta had been "that close" to leaving, "But then there was the congregation and the children – that's what made me stay."

A room of one's own

Several of the women nevertheless managed to find "rooms of their own" within the parameters of marriage. A door that could be closed and a separate bed became a way to make their own decisions about their bodies and their time. Elina described mutual irritation in the shared bedroom, though she was the one who had to adapt. "You were supposed to get up early and go to bed early." As soon as there was enough space, she moved to a bedroom of her own. "I remember thinking, 'Now I'll turn off the light whenever I please.'"

The move, or flight, from a shared bedroom might be a reaction to lack of communication or sexual dominance and sometimes occurred against the husband's will. When the couple was not in agreement about the change, it became the women's task to hide this break with convention from outsiders. The husband continued sleeping in the couple's double bed while the wife found somewhere else to sleep. "The first place we lived I slept on a cot; at the next place, in an alcove; in our last house in a hall leading to his room. I couldn't stand sharing a bedroom," related Greta, who finally moved to her own apartment, though without divorcing. Now she was both "alone and part of a couple," but more on her own terms. She was happy about the independence that having her own mailbox symbolized and about living alone. "It wasn't life in the fast lane, but at least I could be by myself." In Irina's marriage, on the other hand, there was never any disagreement: husband and wife shared a desire for separate bedrooms, and once the children had moved out and there was enough space they could arrange things that way.

Friendships

Family and kinship networks – and for many, paid employment – took most of the women's time and attention, but they had other social contacts as well. Friends were important, both their own and those shared with other family members, although opportunities for interaction varied over the years. Some women had felt free to pursue contacts outside the home and to invite people over. "Without a woman friend you'd go crazy," said Signe. Gertrud had also felt no constraints about getting together with others. "We've been quite unique, the two of us, doing things our own way. He says I should feel free to go out." At the same time many women felt that their personal friendships had to take a back seat to the needs and demands of husbands, children, and extended family. Sara felt she had failed both herself and her friends after she married. "It was my own fault I lost contact with the old crowd."

Some women felt isolated because their husbands were opposed to having visitors or disapproved of their wives having contacts of their own outside the family. "I longed to get out all through the marriage," said Blenda, who had remarried later in life. She was accustomed to socializing with family and friends, but now found herself shut in with a man who neither wanted to go out nor have guests. It became difficult to leave him at home or to break the unspoken social rule of "doing things as a couple." After his death, in the last ten years of her life, she was glad to once again be able to have a social life on her own terms. Linnea also felt her husband kept her under surveillance: if he saw her having a good time with others, he insisted they both go home.

Over time, some of the women in unhappy marriages had been more likely to follow their own inclinations. "I went to a meeting when I couldn't stand being at home. I told him I was old now and he shouldn't interfere," related Elina. Greta also found interests outside the home in order to stay sane. "My husband says I'm running away, and I am. It's a way for me to survive."

Social relationships

Malin, who had just lost her husband, mentioned a disparity she had noticed in her circle of friends. "I don't think older women are held in much regard," she said. "If the wife dies before the husband, he's invited everywhere, but if the wife is alone it's as if she's completely forgotten." Signe described a similar experience. After her husband's death, visits from her female friends were less frequent because their husbands no longer wanted to come along. "But why didn't they come by themselves?" she exclaimed in frustration.

Vera also mentioned that a woman living alone received few invitations. "Single women are segregated – we're supposed to socialize with each other." She noticed that she was not invited to the same events as her married friends and was convinced the reason had nothing to do with interests or preferred topics of conversation. She was accustomed to interacting with men at work and enjoyed their company. "But you end up with groups of women, not with couples," she stated. In a circle of friends she might also feel isolated if discussion was dominated by topics that were outside her personal experience. Colleagues she met in her free time did not talk about their jobs but about husbands and children. Similarly, Britt-Marie longed for a friend who "didn't always have a thousand things she had to consider first." All her friends were married with children. When grandchildren were the main topic of conversation despite everyone knowing she had none, Karin felt invisible and left out.

When Elina came to Sweden from war-torn Finland, she faced a particular kind of alienation. She carried within her painful experiences that native Swedes did not understand, and many seemed uninterested in what she had gone through. The language barrier also cut her off and made her lonely. "I wanted to be with people a lot but I couldn't really talk." The situation was exacerbated because her husband, though born in Sweden, spoke only Finnish himself and was not integrated into Swedish society. Irina, who came to Sweden as a refugee from Hungary in the 1950s, had an entirely different experience. She described the warm welcome her family received and felt this period was a high point in her life. A partial explanation for the discrepancy in the women's responses may be their different social classes. Elina had little education, knew no foreign languages and had married a working-class man, whereas Irina had studied several languages, was able to learn Swedish quickly and was married to a highly educated man who was immediately sought after in the Swedish work force.

Organizational life

Many of the women had joined organizations or taken courses. They had sung in choirs, played musical instruments, danced, exercised, gone swimming, read books, learned new languages, or taken up weaving and embroidery, and felt that these various activities expanded their horizons and helped them learn new things and make new friends. In organizational life their assigned tasks ranged from making coffee and arranging parties to raising money or serving on the board of directors. Small, local organizations were especially important opportunities to meet others. Here the women could find pleasure in being useful. Often they did handiwork that was sold to support charitable causes.

Gertrud was nevertheless disappointed in the "couples mentality" that dominated in the pensioners' association she had joined, despite the fact that most members were women. To have any influence in the organization a woman not only had to be married, she also needed to establish a public profile alongside her husband. "Everyone appears in couples," she said, but her husband was neither willing nor able to participate, which gave her lower status and less authority than other married women. Since male dominance was a factor in organizational life, women's organizations were particularly appealing to Sara. "Women shared many experiences and recognized this in each other without talking much about it," she said. "You can get away from discrimination and the sense that you're not valued as highly." But even in an organization that worked to promote women's rights, she occasionally encountered opposition, including from women who experienced her efforts as calling into question their own choices in life.

Political engagement

A number of the women became involved in human rights issues, both at home and abroad. Signe, the mother of ten, worked to promote peace and participated in various protest demonstrations. "I wanted to do something to prevent war," she said. As a district nurse, Greta came into contact with women who had been abused. Her own experience of psychological abuse motivated her to help establish several women's shelters in the area where she lived. She herself not only responded to phone calls from women in distress, she often became personally involved in helping them; an alternative place to live might be in her own home. She sometimes stayed overnight with women who felt threatened and afraid, and as a result received threatening phone calls herself.

After a visit to Africa, the artist Marta became involved in establishing a school for handicrafts to enable women to support themselves and their children. For several years she put her own work aside in order to raise money for the school. The effort was successful but took a toll on her personal finances; as a result she was forced to move to a smaller, less expensive apartment that doubled as her studio.

Some of the women had been active in politics. In Vera's opinion, women could be especially effective when it came to housing and social issues. She stressed how important it had been for her personally that she could make her voice heard and that her efforts were appreciated, but she also recalled that a woman's position could be difficult because the men stuck together, proposing each other for committee assignments. One incident she remembered as particularly offensive. During the nomination process, a man had pronounced her unworthy of a political post because she was unmarried. No one had protested.

Care of ailing husbands

Several of the married women had cared for their husbands when they were seriously ill. Those who also worked outside the home described having great difficulty focusing on their jobs. They also felt the healthcare system was predicated on their involvement, especially if they had medical training. "I was working, but was afraid to leave home," said Frida, who was a nurse. She saw no real possibility of escaping responsibility for her husband's care. When he refused hospital treatment for a lung condition because he had such faith in her, she felt powerless and vulnerable. "Having someone at home who might suffocate meant I hardly dared sleep at night. When I was at work I'd wonder whether he'd be lying dead on the floor when I got home." She did not think the medical profession was aware of or acknowledged her efforts. One of the aftereffects of caring for her husband was an injured arm muscle that did not heal properly.

Gertrud, who was also a nurse, thought it fell to her to assume responsibility for her husband's rehabilitation after a heart attack. She described her growing anxiety and alarm when she did not succeed in making him quit smoking. Others noted that their attempts at teaching their husbands a healthier lifestyle intensified after the men had been ill. Often the effort had not been gratifying. "He refused to eat healthy food – he never got past adolescence," as Sara put it.

Two of the women were married to men who suffered periodic bouts of depression. During such periods, Greta, the minister's wife, took over most of the parish work, in the office, with confirmation pupils, and so on. It was also up to her to arrange for a substitute preacher when her husband was hospitalized. His tendency to place blame on her intensified during these periods: "He'd harp on things, over and over, to somehow make me look like a sinner. I was in despair!" If she was away from home he might draw attention to his neediness by threatening suicide. She realized he was ill and felt sympathy for him, but she was also furious about the constraints and the burden of guilt brought on by his behavior.

Malin's husband also suffered periods of depression, during which she always worried he would quit his job. By talking to him encouragingly, she tried to help him overcome his low spirits and remain at work. "You can't let him down. If you do, you're not a good wife," she said. Throughout the marriage she had seen herself as the primary breadwinner in the family.

A number of the women had provided home care for elderly husbands who were ill. Several were themselves around 80 years old and not in good health. The women described heavy lifting, sleep disturbances and exhaustion. For most of them, the most strenuous aspect of caregiving was never being able to rest for an extended period and being forced out of bed several times a night to attend to various needs. Not caring for their husbands was still out of the question, even for those whose marriages were deeply unhappy. "I can imagine how it is for him – that's my fate. I'd rather suffer myself than let them drag him away by force," said Valborg when her husband, who needed around-the-clock care, refused to move to a care facility. Sometimes her efforts were beyond what was actually called for. Her husband had been issued a toilet pail that he expected her to empty despite the fact that he could walk to the bathroom. "He takes advantage of me, you see," she said. Most difficult of all was that he never showed any appreciation. "You do everything you can for him and then he's just aggressive and impossible." For a long time she was on the verge of collapse. "Last night I lay awake wondering how I'd get through. I want to die!" she burst out at one interview.

The women were extremely tied down. They could only leave home very briefly and could virtually never travel. Often it was up to them to arrange for another caregiver or someone to "look in on" the husband when they needed to run errands or go to the doctor themselves. "I felt so trapped," said Klary, who was the sole caregiver for her handicapped husband for more than ten years. She wanted to care for him, but also to be able to get away occasionally, if only for a walk. That made her husband anxious. "He'd look at the clock when I left and again when I came back." Others told similar stories. Leaving the invalid husband alone for an hour or a day created such tension that freedom was seldom worth the price.

The women were also responsible for giving their husbands medication and shots, changing bandages and assisting with personal hygiene. Klary's husband, a diabetic, needed daily insulin injections and regular mealtimes. He also had a catheter with a urine bag that needed to be changed every morning. The work was also physically strenuous for Klary. "It was hard to get his wheelchair into the bathroom and to get him in and out of bed I had to lift him." The result was that she injured a shoulder. "He was heavy, despite being thin," she said. Unlike Valborg, however, Klary received recognition from her husband. "It's a good thing you're so capable," he had said. Even so, she wondered how things would have been if *she* had been ill. "Don't think it would have been so great if I'd been bedridden and he had to take care of me. He'd probably have been cross."

Eventually most of the women had no choice but to give up their caregiving responsibilities. No matter how worn out they were, this made them feel they had let their husbands down; after all, the men did not want institutional care. The women nevertheless continued to be involved in their husbands' care through daily visits and by seeing to it that they got the attention they needed. As long as they were able, they also brought their husbands home to visit.

In retrospect

For couples who were close and loved each other, the sense of connection continued into old age. After retirement, some husbands helped their wives by taking on practical tasks in the home in ways that previously had been unimaginable. "He was really capable," Klary related. "He cleaned, washed clothes, had dinner ready when I came home. It was wonderful. I was tired when I got home from work." Once both husband and wife had retired, however, in most cases the division of labor and caregiving responsibilities reverted to old patterns.

A number of the women were widows when we interviewed them. "His picture is always beside me when I go to bed. I say goodnight and then good morning," said Malin. She mourned her husband and tried to maintain a sense of closeness. She and others missed the shared daily routines and reflected on all the things they could have done together if their husbands had been alive and well. In their thoughts, they also tried to make peace with aspects of the marriage that had not been satisfying.

Others found it difficult to think back on their marriages, and our interviews also brought out things that had been forgotten. Elina had "tried to repress" raw and painful memories. At the time of the interviews Valborg had given up; she no longer expected so much as a kind word from her husband. Some time later, when he died without them having a chance to talk things over, this became the most devastating memory of all. Her hope of finding reconciliation and a bond, perhaps even a little love, was now conclusively eradicated. The minister's wife Greta likewise found it difficult to think about the past.

Several of the women mourned a love they had never found. Blenda had been suspicious of men after divorcing an alcoholic. When she eventually remarried, she did not find what she longed for with that husband, either. "He was faithful," she said. "But I miss not having met someone I could really love."

3

Childbearing

A social issue

Fifteen of the twenty women had borne children between the mid-1930s and the mid-1960s, a period that coincided with major changes in society's concern about childbearing (Forssén 2012). At the beginning of the period, there was still great ignorance about pregnancy and giving birth and circumstances varied depending on social class and marital status. Toward the end of the 1930s the issue of access to contraceptives once again came to the fore, leading in the late 1930s to a lift of the ban on their sale. Sexual activity outside marriage was still condemned by many, but the availability of legal contraceptives was expected to protect women from the strain of too-frequent pregnancies and to reduce the economic burden in families that already had many children.[8] At around the same time the first law permitting abortion – albeit on narrowly defined grounds, primarily medical – went into effect. Non-medical grounds were initially not taken into account and later were considered only to a limited degree. Consequently the number of illegal abortions continued to be high. As late as the mid-1940s, certain large urban hospitals had special wards for women who needed care after illegal abortions. After 1945, when penicillin came into use, the mortality rate declined, but the aftereffects were often serious, especially for impoverished women; those from middle and upper-class backgrounds were often better able to arrange for a medically safe procedure. The

---

8 A leader in these questions was the newly established National Association for Sexual Education, headed by the well-known sex educator Elise Ottesen-Jensen. She and others made extensive tours of the country lecturing to both women and men. The mission was to provide information about sexual reproduction and how to protect oneself from pregnancy. Another message was that love between human beings should be valued and treated with respect. Women were also fitted for diaphragms under somewhat primitive conditions (see Thorgren 2011).

abortion issue, like many other health matters, was thus a class issue. The number of illegal abortions remained high until the 1960s, when the law began to be less strictly applied. Since 1975 women in Sweden have had the right to make their own decision about abortion until the eighteenth week of pregnancy. After that period permission is required from the National Board of Health and Welfare.

Changes in Swedish legislation during this same period nevertheless obstructed the rights of certain women with regard to sexuality and reproduction. A 1934 law, expanded in 1941, authorized sterilization without consent for reasons of "insanity, feeble-mindedness or an aberrant way of life" (*Norstedts uppslagsbok* 1962). Many women were sterilized against their will, often without even being informed about the nature of the operation. Those suffering from psychological disorders, the poor, and women from the Roma and Sami minorities were the primary targets.[9] Forced sterilization essentially ended in the 1960s but the law was repealed only in 1976.

Female physicians were among those who had called for subsidies to pregnant women early in the century. In the early 1930s women who could establish need received a sum to outfit the newborn baby. In the 1950s this support was extended to all new mothers. The 1930s also brought the first state-sponsored maternity leave, with the right to 30 days of paid leave for women in the work force. This was expanded to three months in the 1950s.[10] Single mothers, however, still faced major obstacles, both financial and social, and their children also experienced shame and humiliation. The term "illegitimate" remained in common use during this period. Only in 1970 did these children receive the right to inherit from their fathers.

During the period when participants in the study were having babies a nationwide system of cost-free prenatal clinics and children's clinics was under development, motivated by the low birth rate and high mortality rates for new mothers and infants. In contemporary medical literature, the high mortality rates were largely attributed to the childbearing women themselves, who were depicted as mentally unbalanced and ignorant (see Forssén 2012). Hence prenatal care was judged important in order to educate women and identify risks. Initially, however, many women were unaccustomed to the healthcare system's new involvement with pregnancy and stayed away, which healthcare personnel considered negligent (Jansson 2008: 64). Prenatal

---

9 Since 2000, the rights of certain minority groups, among them the Jews, the Roma, and the Sami, have been protected under Swedish law.
10 Since then, the right to time off in connection with the birth of a child has successively expanded (see Chapter 11).

clinics were (and are) run by midwives, with a chief physician as consultant.[11]

Getting pregnant

The women's fear of becoming pregnant before marriage was readily apparent in the interviews. "Having sex before the wedding was out of the question," as one of them put it. Elna, who lived in a rural area, recalled the overwhelming sense of shame her premarital pregnancy caused. She was afraid to go out and pulled her corset so tight that she could scarcely breathe. More than fifty years later she could awaken from a nightmare in which, overcome by disgrace, she gave birth to a child.

As previously mentioned, sexuality and the intimate side of married life were difficult topics to bring up in interviews. Many of the women were reluctant to discuss methods of contraception, although *coitus interruptus*, "the usual thing – not reaching the finishing line," and condom use were often implied. The problem with these methods was that women were dependent on their husbands' cooperation, as Greta, the midwife, learned. When she could not understand why she suddenly felt queasy one day, her husband confessed that he had only pretended to use a condom. In her work Greta encountered many women whose babies were unplanned.

Some of the married women lived in fear of becoming pregnant throughout their fertile years. This was the case for Signe, who had nine children by the age of thirty-one. She lived in an area where contraceptives, although no longer banned, were not generally available, and there was no information about them from healthcare providers. "I'd never heard of or seen a condom," she related. At first she thought breast-feeding would protect her from pregnancy, and her husband also tried to "be careful." "I got pregnant anyway," she said. "I hadn't even gotten my period back." Sometimes Signe felt she had been "born to have babies." When she became pregnant for the tenth time after a six-year hiatus, it was difficult starting over. She felt her life had improved once her youngest daughter was older and past the "dirty diaper stage."

Even well educated women were poorly informed. Although Sara studied biology at university, she was initially entirely unfamiliar with contraceptives and the workings of her body, nor did Gertrud, a nurse,

---

[11] Eventually virtually all Swedish women received prenatal care and medical attention during labor and delivery, which has contributed to the current low maternal and infant mortality rate.

know much about how to protect herself from pregnancy. Both had unplanned babies early in marriage, Sara while still a student. Only then did she "figure out what contraceptives were all about" and get a diaphragm. The first two children of Linnea, the physician, were also unplanned.

Britt Marie, the youngest of the women and a city-dweller, had never lived with a man but did have an active sex life. She described being "incredibly grateful" that she had learned to use a diaphragm, and had later tried birth control pills, available in Sweden from the mid-1960s. "It was fantastic," she said, "to be able to have sex without risking pregnancy!" In the 1960s, the IUD also became available in Sweden.

A number of the women indicated that they had viewed pregnancy as determined by fate. If they married, they might have children – this was something they could neither plan nor control. Even Malin, who had a strong professional identity, let chance determine her childbearing. "In those days that's the way it was," she said. "Things just took their own course." Estrid, who referred to her "five hostages of fortune," felt the same way.

A couple of the women with one or two children would have liked to have more, but for varying reasons were not able. Karin had a traumatic experience in connection with the birth of her second child and after finally recovering did not become pregnant again. Elina suffered repeated miscarriages and was childless for many years. Her fifth pregnancy produced a baby that died shortly after birth. On the sixth attempt she finally gave birth to a baby that survived, but after that she was physically and emotionally exhausted. Frida remained childless despite having sought medical help early in marriage.

None of the women described having an illegal abortion, but Irina from Hungary had had a legal one. Under the communist regime, there was a brief period when women could freely choose abortion as long as they had already borne three children.

Some women appeared to have taken control of reproduction from the start. Edit related, "We had plans that we followed. Then we thought it was time for a baby, and it happened almost right away. They are real love babies!" Klary and her husband were instead in agreement that they did *not* want children; they wanted to be free. They used condoms for protection. It is thus apparent that in marriages where husband and wife had a good relationship and made decisions jointly it was possible, to some extent, to plan childbearing.

The single women who had not borne children had made their peace with that outcome, though they might sometimes feel they had missed something or grieve about the necessity of making a choice. But as

Marta said, "There have been so many children in my life anyway – schoolchildren, nieces and nephews, all the children I've painted. You don't have to give birth to them yourself."

At the prenatal clinic

In the interviews, the women dwelled more than anticipated on their pregnancies and deliveries, and their memories were detailed and precise. Valborg, for instance, related that forty years earlier she had started bleeding in gestational week thirty-one when expecting her third child: "I think it was on a Saturday – no, it was Friday night when I started bleeding. We were expecting company. My sister-in-law was coming with her twins. And I had bought a chicken that I needed to fry up…" Edit described one of her deliveries by specifying exact times. "It was twelve noon when we went to the hospital, and she was born at six that evening. It was on a Friday."

The detailed recollections of the women also included their encounters with the medical establishment. During this period, when prenatal care was being expanded in Sweden, a number of the women were caught between the old system, where women managed pregnancy and babies on their own, and the new order in which the healthcare system was highly involved. Their background and circumstances determined the degree to which they took part in new developments. Those who were used to getting by independently when prenatal care was not readily available, among them rural-dwelling Signe, did not contact medical personnel until late in their pregnancies even after access improved. Signe's experience, moreover, was that it was hard to make her voice heard in the prenatal care system. In her ninth pregnancy the physician declared she would have twins. "Not a chance," Signe had said. "I've had eight children and I'd notice if something different." This made the doctor "cross" – he "couldn't take it" that she disagreed with him – and the midwife followed the doctor's lead in her preparations. But no twins came. During her next pregnancy Signe waited even longer before seeking medical attention despite being unusually tired. On arrival at the clinic she was found to be anemic, and the delivery was complicated. The midwife rebuked her: "'Well, things nearly went very badly this time. Now you see what can happen when you don't have checkups.' So she really told me off!" Estrid, living in a large city, told a similar story of being reproved by the consultant doctor when attending the clinic for the first time late in her fourth pregnancy.

Since Elna wanted to do the right thing she visited the prenatal clinic early in her second pregnancy. No one there believed she was pregnant.

When it eventually became clear that she was, her constant nausea was dismissed as a bagatelle. "The doctor said, 'Just have a piece of toast in the morning.' I said, 'But it's not just in the morning – it goes on all day.'" She continued to vomit throughout the pregnancy; toward the end she was diagnosed as suffering from malnutrition.

Linnea, who was a gynecologist herself, realized early in her second pregnancy that something was wrong and noticed that amniotic fluid was seeping out. But no one believed her. A male colleague dismissed her observations with the words, "It's probably just a little urine leaking." When she went into premature labor it was discovered that she had been expecting twins, one of whom had died much earlier.

Clearly the new prenatal clinics did not always provide the support women needed and expected. Most notably, there was little allowance for their own experience of and thoughts about their pregnancies. A hierarchical medical care system run by specialists had taken over a field of knowledge that many women previously had considered their own.

Heavy work during pregnancy

Most of the women had continued working as before throughout pregnancy. Neither the women themselves nor those around them gave special consideration to their condition. Often they had demanding work tasks both inside and outside the home. Estrid, a cleaner at construction sites, had two miscarriages she blamed on her job. "I must have lifted something that was too heavy," she said. Seeking medical attention afterward seemed pointless.

Gertrud, who was a nurse, wanted to continue working after she became pregnant, but neither her older colleagues nor her employer "took kindly" to this. "It wasn't the usual practice for nurses to keep their jobs when they started a family." For this reason it was important to demonstrate that she could still work at full capacity. In retrospect she thought she had been foolish. "All those heavy, anesthetized patients who had to be lifted from a trolley into bed. It was tough." By evening she was utterly exhausted. "But I was healthy, after all, so there was no reason to call in sick."

Except during the last of her ten pregnancies, Signe had often felt stronger than usual when she was expecting; heavy menstrual bleeding made her anemic between pregnancies. "You're always tired and queasy at first, but after that I was stronger than ever before. Good Lord, how I could work!" Toward the end of a pregnancy, however, she was worn out, while simultaneously needing to make arrangements for being away from home. She had to take care of the baking, cleaning, and laundry, and recalled how exhausting this was. Once, shortly before giving birth, she had hauled the laundry across the ice from the island where she lived to the mainland. After climbing over snowdrifts with the heavy laundry basket, she remained sitting for a long time without the energy to go on. "I thought, good God, I can't move. This is where I'll have the baby – I'll just stay here till it comes."

Valborg had continued with heavy farm work for several days after her amniotic fluid began leaking. "I was out putting hay on the drying racks and strained myself so the water broke." She had no idea this could endanger the baby, and no one around her reacted. The baby was in breach position and died during delivery. "The midwife and the doctor were angry with me: 'How could you do such a thing, Mrs. Johansson?' they said. And I started asking myself the same thing: How could I?!"

For Signe and Valborg, whose work was unpaid but physically demanding, it was expected as a matter of course that they would continue as usual until they gave birth. Women who became pregnant when somewhat older also found it draining. Anna, who was past forty, had back problems from many years of farm labor and was bedridden for much of her fourth pregnancy. A late pregnancy was also the reason Linnea did not follow through on the divorce that had been on her mind for years. She remembered the overwhelming exhaustion in the evenings that made her think, "I couldn't move from the spot if the house were on fire."

Preparing for childbirth

Though hospital care soon became the norm for everyone, several of the older women in the study, in particular those who lived in rural areas, had given birth to their first children at home. Knowledge about the process of labor and delivery varied considerably among the women and consequently their preparation and planning also differed. Signe was always very aware of when the baby was due. She knew when she had had intercourse with her husband, who was often away during the week, and could calculate on that basis. "I had no intention of going to the hospital until the very last minute," she said.

Others were less prepared for what lay ahead. Sara, still a university student when pregnant the first time, had no idea when the baby was due. "I knew I was pregnant, of course, but the due date..." Nor did she know what would happen during labor and delivery, since no one had provided the relevant information. Her mother had recently died and at the prenatal clinic no one addressed the subject. She had tried to read up on her own, but this did not prove helpful. Giving birth came as a shock to her.

For Irina in Hungary, the abnormal circumstances of World War II determined her experience of childbirth. The first time, she related, "An alarm had gone off and sirens were blaring when we went to the hospital. My mother was with me. My husband and my father were both in military service." When her second child was due she chose to give birth at home because the food at the hospital was substandard. The war was over when her third child was born, but in a climate of political persecution her husband had been arrested.

Economic factors were also significant. Edit could choose to give birth at a private hospital near her home. "There was no public hospital nearby and you might have a long drive. My husband wouldn't accept that," she related. Others described walking long distances well after labor pains had begun. Elna, pregnant for the third time, had moved to the city shortly before – now without a partner since her husband had asked for a divorce. "It was a long walk across town. My landlady went with me. The contractions just kept coming, harder and harder, and I walked as fast as I could." Estrid, who had also walked to the hospital, gave a concise explanation: "I couldn't afford a taxi."

Most of the women had given birth to their children before the 1960s, when it became more common for fathers to be present during labor and delivery.

Pain during childbirth

Pain relief during childbirth was a frequent topic of discussion in the middle of the previous century. The British physician Dr. Grantly Dick-Read (1993) regarded labor pain as a consequence of civilization and changing social ideals regarding womanhood. His view that modern women ought to recapture their "natural ability" to give birth without pain became internationally influential and was adopted by many physicians and midwives. In Sweden, "natural delivery" implied that doctors should not interfere, and pain alleviation techniques were introduced late. Nitrous oxide gas ("laughing gas") was the only method in use until the 1960s, but was not available at all hospitals (see Forssén 2012). Midwives took responsibility for home births as well as for hospital deliveries; doctors became involved only if complications occurred. These are still the Swedish guidelines.

Some of the women described their experience of childbirth in positive terms. On her own initiative, Estrid had done relaxation exercises during pregnancy after reading about the technique in *Reader's Digest*. She thought it worked well and made her labor easy. Edit, who also thought things had gone "very well," recalled that she had been given "a little whiff of ether." Malin did not experience any "difficulties or complications" and also praised the care she had received on the maternity ward. "In those days the care you got was excellent – you were pampered. The midwife and nursing staff came and made your bed."[12]

Others, in contrast, recalled childbirth as the most painful experience of their lives. "It was the worst thing I've ever been through, and back then there was no laughing gas or anything else," said Sara. Signe also found it strenuous to give birth. With a touch of irony, she summarized her experience with "Babies aren't exactly attached to you on the outside."

A number of women described feeling abandoned during labor, as contractions went on hour after hour without anyone else in the room. "No one paid you any mind – you just had to grit your teeth and bear it," Sara remembered. Several women were not taken seriously when they told the staff that the baby would come soon and described their fear that no one would be there to help. Elna, who already had two children, knew she had reached the pushing stage but was told she had come to the clinic too early and would be dealt with later. Shortly thereafter, she managed to get attention at the very last minute before the baby was born. "I rang the bell over and over – the midwife only had time to put on one glove before my daughter came out."

The women had often encountered the attitude that childbirth is supposed to be painful. Elna had asked why and been told, "That's why you love your children." A male physician had also told her that "women always tolerate pain better." She continued, "It's as if they count on that – it's up to you to get through it as best you can." Anyone who was not patient and silent risked criticism or reprimand. Valborg was told she was "a silly whiner" when she cried out in pain during her first labor. The next time she fought hard not to moan, despite the fact that the baby's position was wrong and the midwife pressed down hard on her belly to get it out. She did not want to be called a whiner again.

---

12 Until the mid-1960s women were expected to remain in bed for at least a week after giving birth, that is, during their entire stay on the maternity ward. Nowadays most women stay just one or two days and are told to be up and about again a few hours after giving birth.

Many women had vaginal tears toward the end of labor or underwent an episiotomy. At the time it was customary to put in stitches without administering anesthesia. When she protested, Elna was considered uncooperative and demanding. "I said it hurt. 'But you just popped out a baby like it was nothing – this can't be such a big deal'" was the response. "It was just awful, lying there holding your breath while they sewed you up." Elna and several others received stitches made of what they called "barbed wire," a kind of steel thread that when clipped made little barbs that were very painful. They also made it difficult to sit. "It was a year before I could sit properly and for several months it was hard to pee. We had a wooden barrel. I put rubber around the edge so I could sit."

A traumatic experience

Karin's second delivery was difficult and prolonged, but this was not what remained on her mind. It was what followed that left an indelible memory. She needed stitches, but no anesthesia was planned. When she protested strenuously, her request for it was granted "as a favor, as they put it." Karin continued: "So they shouted for the doctor who was supposed to do it. I'll never forget when he entered the room, without a white coat. He was wearing a brown suit. I was tremendously upset ... and I think he smelled like smoke – but never mind about that. But he wasn't wearing a white coat! It was at night ... I was distraught at the time and I've never forgotten it." Karin associated her distress at breastfeeding and strange bodily symptoms and "dreams" with this disturbing event: "I must have had a real shock then," she concluded, describing her anguish and quaking when feeding time approached, making breastfeeding "a horrible experience" for her. When she lay down after nursing she felt as if she were losing consciousness and was terrified she would never wake up. It took her more than a year to recover from her symptoms. Thinking she was the only one who was "so strange" and did not enjoy breastfeeding, Karin did not share her experiences with anyone. It was fifty years before she broke her silence, telling her story for the first time in an interview for this study.

Other women also felt isolated after traumatic experiences in childbirth and wished they had been able to talk to someone who could empathize with their situation. Elina, whose baby died a few days after birth, was given no information whatsoever about the cause of death and did not have the strength to ask. Only after returning home did she, at her own request, receive instructions about how to inhibit milk production. Blenda had undergone a difficult forceps delivery and was running a high fever afterward. Since the baby had been moved to a children's hospital, she was not allowed to see it for many days. She herself was released from the maternity ward before she felt strong enough to manage on her own. She was convinced she was treated so badly because she was in the middle of a divorce.

Valborg had suffered complications during delivery several times. Her first baby came out "limp and blue" with the umbilical cord around its neck. The second baby died, as previously mentioned, after the water broke while she was working in the fields. During her third pregnancy she spent many weeks in the hospital because of bleeding. At the time of the interview she was still preoccupied with the baby that had died during delivery. Ever since she had asked herself over and over why doctors had not performed a cesarean section. A woman in the adjoining bed had pressed for that procedure under similar circumstances, and her baby had survived. At every interview and in every telephone conversation both during and after the interview period, Valborg accused herself vehemently and mourned her child: "I think about it every day, blaming myself. If it hadn't been for my stupidity she would be alive!"

Home again

Several women in the study had objected to the rule of staying in bed for several days after giving birth. Signe thought extended bed rest made her "really tired and weak" and stole all her energy, energy she needed when she returned home to her other children. "You didn't have help at home except when you were in the hospital,[13] so you knew what lay in store," she said. The post-partum period of rest thus ended abruptly; once home again, it was back to the usual routine of housework and childcare. Elna, whose first baby was born at home, was also told to stay in bed for nine days. The minute the midwife left

---

13 Beginning in 1928, Swedish municipalities provided trained "home helpers" to assist families with children, for instance when the mother was in the hospital after giving birth. Until the 1960s, municipal boards determined who had the right to such assistance, so criteria varied from place to place. Subsequently, so-called "home samaritans," who ordinarily assisted the elderly, might help families in certain cases. The assumption today is that the father will be at home – by law, new fathers are guaranteed ten days of paid vacation time – or that grandparents or other close relatives will help out if necessary.

she got up. "There were lots of things I felt I needed to do. Actually, I hardly stayed in bed at all."

Karin recalled the relentless exhaustion that overcame her after the traumatic experience of her second delivery. Laundry or other heavy labor seemed like an insurmountable obstacle and she could feel her usual sense of self-control slipping. "Then I came home. It was so primitive, the laundry and everything. I remember being very, very tired, and often irritated because I was tired."

A number of the women commented on how vital it was to have support from someone close to them. Mothers and mothers-in-law were especially important. "I relied a great deal on what Mom said, much more than I relied on anyone else," said Elna. Those who did not have this help described feeling isolated and anxious. Sara, who had lost her mother just before her first child was born, described how terrified she felt during the first period at home. She knew nothing about babies: "I was scared stiff, thought she'd die. I turned to books since I had to get through this somehow."

Breastfeeding

Only a couple of the women expressed a positive attitude toward breastfeeding. Estrid had felt it was "as natural as life itself" to nurse her babies and continued for a full year. For Irina, who endured food shortages during the war, breastfeeding was equally self-evident. Far more women had mixed or negative feelings: nursing had been unpleasant or painful and had tied them down. These reactions were in stark contrast to the generally accepted belief that breastfeeding was a wonderful experience. During the 1940s and '50s, moreover, nursing was supposed to follow a strict schedule. The baby should be fed every four hours, neither more nor less often, according to the experts.

While still on the maternity ward Sara was scoffed at because she found it painful to breastfeed. "I had to quit before long – I had huge sores on my breasts. It was terribly difficult." Despite her uncontrollable shaking, Karin had continued breastfeeding for the prescribed six months. She, too, had painful eczema on her breasts. "It hurt like crazy when he sucked," she said. On top of that, she had more milk than the baby needed and used a pump to provide milk for a woman who had had twins. "I kept it up all summer long," she said. "They came over to fetch it." Elina, who also had an excess of milk, went to the hospital herself several times a week to donate it. "There was so much milk – it was disgusting."

Elna had nursed her first baby for a full year despite disliking it and continuously longing to quit. "I felt such resistance every time. It didn't hurt, but there was such an unpleasant feeling..." Believing it was best for the baby, she continued nevertheless, though she ignored the four-hour rule from the start, picking up the baby whenever she thought it was called for. After her second baby was born her milk dried up quickly – due to stress, she believed – and she breastfed for only a month. This was exhausting for other reasons since the midwife told her not to bottle-feed. "I sat there trying to feed her with a spoon. It might be two hours before I got it all into her."

The women had kept silent about breastfeeding problems and feelings of discomfort, just as they kept silent about difficult experiences in pregnancy and childbirth. They believed they were the only ones who felt this way and were afraid to be open, even with their closest women friends.

Many also found it tiring to breastfeed. Once Signe had nearly dropped the baby as she started to fall asleep while sitting on the edge of the bed. She was among those who switched to a bottle after only a few months; then her husband could sometimes help out. Anna also thought a bottle was more practical, since someone else could take over if she was away; she had farm animals and a country store to take care of. Before formula was available, however, preparing a bottle was labor-intensive: oat flour had to be boiled, strained, filtered, and thinned.

None of the women with paying jobs breastfed for very long. As noted above, the maternity leave guaranteed by law was short and those who wanted to keep their jobs had to return to work quickly, after which it became difficult to accommodate nursing in the schedule.

4

Caring for Children and Other Family Members

Family policy

At mid-century, the political position on family life reflected the dominant perception in society at large that women who had borne children should care for them themselves. There was essentially no state-sponsored childcare and mothers who worked outside the home had to make their own arrangements by turning to nannies or home daycare providers, help from mothers and other female relatives, or by taking their children along to work. In the 1940s, a proposal from women urging that daycare centers be built was voted down by the male-dominated parliament with the motivation that women's place was in the home and taking care of children was a maternal duty.

To promote healthy child development, free medical checkups were offered at children's clinics and vaccinations were implemented for all children beginning in the late 1930s. After 1948, supplemental payments to families with children provided additional support. A new feature in family finances was that the money was paid out to mothers, not fathers, since this was believed to be a better guarantee that the subsidy would actually benefit the children.[14] For many married women, this sum was the only money they themselves controlled. In the late 1940s women also acquired the right to be their children's legal guardians.

---

14 Child subsidies are still paid to all children in Sweden. The amount has successively increased since the system was introduced and at present also includes a so-called third child supplement: double the amount for the third child and any subsequent children.

Motherhood: a mixed blessing

All the women in our study who had children were glad their lives had included this experience. "Being a mother is wonderful," said Elina, who had gone through six pregnancies but only given birth to one child that survived. But life with children could also bring pain and sorrow. Both Elina and Valborg had lost a baby immediately after birth and an additional three women had gone through the death of an older child. "I haven't felt like singing since my boy died," said Estrid, who lost a son in a moped accident.

Things were difficult for the two women, Blenda and Elna, who were divorced and raised their children alone. Neither of them wanted any contact with the children's father, nor did the fathers make an effort to see the children. In dire straits financially and without access to childcare, Elna was forced to put the baby born shortly after the divorce up for adoption. At the middle of the previous century, this was still a common outcome for women unable to care for their children themselves.[15] That the decision was extremely painful for Elna was clear. She was unable to eat and became ill: "Eventually I was so done in that I fainted on the street." No one except her parents knew of the child's existence.

Signe was left a widow with ten children when the youngest was only a few years old. She, too, had great difficulty supporting them. At one point she asked a government agency to provide firewood, needed for cooking and heating the house. When the request was denied she felt so mortified that she never again requested government assistance.

Some of the women spent long periods caring for others' children: foster children, nieces and nephews, or grandchildren. Among them was Greta, the minister's wife, who served as a foster mother for many years despite having four children of her own. In her position it was virtually a duty to care for children in the parish who had fallen on hard times. The children required time and love; sometimes entire families needed help and support.

Total responsibility

Primary responsibility for children rested on the women. For the two single mothers, this was a given, and both chose to continue living

---

15 Today adoption within Sweden occurs only under exceptional circumstances (for instance the death of the parents) and has been replaced by placement in foster homes or other types of support to families in distress. Almost without exception, children adopted by Swedish parents come from countries outside Europe.

alone with their children, Elna the entire time they were growing up, Blenda until her daughter was a teenager. A number of the married women, both stay-at-home moms and working mothers, viewed it as "natural" and "the right thing" that they took on virtually the entire responsibility for their children. "Mothers and children have always belonged together," said Malin, who despite this attitude always worked outside the home. Others would have liked to share caregiving responsibilities and wished they had more faith in their husbands' capabilities. Several noted how helpless their husbands had been, especially with small babies.

Many fathers were away from home a great deal, often without consulting their wives. If a mother wanted to be away, detailed planning was generally required, and it was by no means certain that the husband would step in to help. Elina recalled an occasion when she asked her husband to watch their daughter and he did not. The daughter was frightened and after that would scarcely leave her mother's side. Linnea's husband, a physician and father of four children, one of them psychologically handicapped, was on call a great deal. "Everyone praised him for taking that on," said Linnea. "But what about his family, then? I was completely alone with the kids all the time!"

Even when they were away from home or in the hospital the women felt responsible for how their children were doing. Signe remembered worrying about having to leave the older ones to fend for themselves when she was on the maternity ward. During her third pregnancy, Valborg had to spend a lengthy period in the hospital. She knew her six-year-old daughter, alone at home with her severely alcoholic husband, was at risk, but no one else was available to care for her.

The sense of responsibility continued while the women were at work. Whenever possible, they called home to check that all was well or to remind their children about various matters. If the children were sick they might run home over the lunch break. When the workday ended there was always a rush to get home.

Availability and vigilance

When the children were small, constant vigilance was necessary. "A mother needs to have her eyes and ears about her at all times," said Signe. The house where her large family lived had neither indoor plumbing nor electricity. The wood-burning stove in the kitchen was almost always hot. Going to the outhouse or into the cellar required careful planning: one child was tied to a piece of furniture, another placed in the woodbin, a third taken along. She cooked with the youngest on her hip; when sewing, a child was always on her lap. If the children were outside she watched them through the window, even if her husband was with them. "You have to have eyes in the back of your head, and men don't." She often had to go outside and call, "But don't you see what's going on?!"

Those with fewer children also felt that taking care of them was "no walk in the park," as Sara put it. She considered her work in the home far more demanding than her paid job as a teacher – never a quiet moment, constantly preoccupied by the children's cries for mommy. Many women also mentioned the necessity of "being available" when the children called, when they came home from school, when they needed help. This close daily contact also made them sensitive to the children's worries and problems, which called for them to listen and offer encouragement and comfort. "They might come to me in the middle of the night, wanting to talk," said Greta. A couple of the women also found it necessary to protect the children from their father. Valborg, for instance, saw to it that her son did not ride in the car when his father was drunk behind the wheel.

It was also important to allow for play. "Everything in its place didn't work for us," said Signe, describing how the children ran around and around in circles, making a mess of the rags she had cut up to make rugs, which she then had to sort out again. Elina often stayed in the bedroom when her daughter was in the living room playing with friends. She saw it as "a breathing spell" and let the children carry on, despite the work cleaning up after them. Linnea held "open house" for children in the neighborhood to help her son make friends.

There were, however, occasions when children were *not* allowed to run wild. Greta, the minister's wife, described what it was like taking the children to church. "Everything was fine until the Creed. At that point the little one had had enough, and that set the others off." From then on her attention was focused on keeping the children in line; only rarely did she get anything out of the service.

Around the clock

The work of being vigilant and available often continued around the clock, and nights could be very short. Signe described early mornings and late evenings. At night the children padded in and wanted to sleep in her bed. "The bed was completely full, from the foot all the way up." Others remembered awakening at the slightest sound, getting up many times each night, going in to check on the children's breathing. Linnea, whose son was hyperactive, described locks on doors, tying down the bed, and constant vigilance to keep him from sneaking out. This continued, night and day, for five years before she could leave him unattended. "I was utterly done in physically from taking care of him," she said. Anna, who got up every morning at 4:30 to milk the cows, was grateful her children were not "night whiners." She did not think she could have managed if they had been.

A child's illness brought even more sleep disruptions. "You were on edge all night long, listening with one ear." Serious illness caused worry as well. Women who had gone through the death of a child felt anxious at the slightest sign that something was wrong. Later in life, this applied to grandchildren as well. Even when a woman herself was ill, primary concern was for the children; she hoped she would have the strength to go on for their sake.

Sleep disturbances might also be an issue when the children were teenagers and out late in the evening; the women might lie awake until they came home. At other times the house was full of young people until late at night. Elina preferred that her daughter invite friends to their place rather than hanging out with a group she did not know. It was difficult, however, to see to it that her husband's sleep was not disturbed, and mornings were hard as well. "I was so tired I scarcely knew my own name," she said.

Training and education

During the 1940s and '50s, the period when most of the women had small children, there was a concerted effort in Sweden to provide expert advice on childcare and childrearing. Some women followed this advice faithfully, especially those who did not have mothers or other experienced women to turn to. "I'm a typical product of the times," said Sara. "Early potty training, cellulose diapers, and a strict schedule." Others trusted their own judgment and capabilities. Signe was among those who most strongly resisted the opinions and admonitions of experts. "How you should handle them varies so much from child to child," she said.

Some believed that girls and boys should be brought up the same way. "I felt strongly about resisting male and female roles," said Gertrud, who was influenced by the incipient social debate about gender equality. Others, like Signe, were more likely to follow the patterns they themselves had grown up with. "The girls had to help with the dishes, not the boys," she said.

It was also essential to teach the children in a broader sense: to give them access to culture, activities, and an education. At home many read aloud to their children or made music with them. To Linnea, it was especially important to help her handicapped son develop language skills. She talked to him continuously and sang a great deal. After three and a half years she reached her goal: he had learned to talk. Women with limited financial resources also tried to provide stimulation and find activities for their children. Blenda bought books for her daughter although this was really beyond her budget, and Elna made an effort to find any kind of entertainment that was free of charge: "I dragged the kids to parks and museums all over town." A great deal of attention was also paid to the children's schooling. The women discussed what had happened in school with them and helped with homework if they were able. They also tried to meet the school's expectations about schedule changes, parent-teacher conferences, acquiring sports equipment, preparing for excursions and so on, which was often difficult time-wise as well as financially. Gertrud and her husband volunteered to chaperone school dances. "It was important for parents to be there," she said. "It was easy to buy beer, and things could get out of hand."

The childcare question

As previously noted, during the 1940s and '50s the predominant attitude was that women with children should not be in the work force, and a number of women in the study expressed delight that they had been able to stay home when their children were small. For those with paying jobs or seeking employment outside the home, the availability of childcare was a determining factor. Subsidized childcare, found primarily in large cities, was extremely limited and designed primarily for single mothers. But there were no places for babies. For as long as possible, Elna tried to manage by bringing her newborn daughter to work, but within a few months had to put the baby up for adoption. She left the two older children alone at home, locked in with enough food to get through the day. Later, when she moved back to her home district, her parents helped with childcare. The practical and emotional support they provided made Elna feel she was better off than many other mothers, whether single or married. With her own mother nearby she could also get advice in matters concerning the children. "She showed me what to do, helped out, gave me self-confidence."

   Blenda managed to solve the childcare problem by taking a position as a maid. Her daughter could be with her all day, and since the two of them lived in her employer's kitchen, her housing situation was also resolved.

Several of the married women who needed paid employment to make ends meet were unable to work because there was no one to watch their children. Estrid did manage, however, to arrange for the children to be with her at the construction site where she worked as a cleaner. In the morning they were asleep when she left. After a few hours she hurried home, fed them and took them along to work. "They had a lot of fun there," she said, "but it wasn't really a safe place for kids."

Although Sara, the teacher, was one of the few who managed to place her children in daycare, things were still not easy. She felt "wretched" when she left them behind, weeping, and hurried off to work, a reaction reinforced by the fact that she was the only woman she knew who did not follow the norm of staying home with the children: "None of the other wives left their kids in daycare."

Women who earned a good salary were able to employ nannies or maids, but there was no way to know whether they were taking good care of the children. Sometimes they suspected that all was not well. Malin said that her "heart nearly broke" when she had to leave although the children wanted her to stay. She remembered her daughter's words as she went down the stairs one morning: "Please, Mommy, stay home with us, just for today!" It was difficult even when the children were older and could manage on their own. Neither Malin nor Sara had dared ask their adult children about their years as "latch-key kids."

Linnea, the physician, was never able to find childcare that would accommodate the needs of her handicapped son. Reluctantly, she stayed home for fifteen years before returning to her profession.

Self-reproach and censure

Despite a constant effort to "be there" for the children, many women felt they could have done more. "Of course you felt inadequate almost all the time," said Sara. "You always had a bad conscience – I think all mothers do," said Elina. None of the women experienced their husbands as having similar guilt feelings. Instead, Elna herself felt guilty for having "given the children a father who didn't care." At the same time she was aware, not least through ongoing social debate, that "children need a father," a conflict she could not resolve. Throughout her life she was tormented by thoughts of the child she had been forced to put up for adoption. At the time of our interviews, she was still asking herself, "Shouldn't I have been able to manage it?"

Some women felt they had already "failed" at breastfeeding and connected this to the children's subsequent eating problems. Elna agonized over the possibility that her smoking was "contagious." Others were worried that they had demanded too much of their children. Those who had continued working outside the home felt they had not spent enough time with their children, even if they had devoted every free moment to them. Such feelings might surface even if work for pay was an economic necessity. "I couldn't resolve the dilemma – I haven't lived in accordance with my belief that mothers should be home with their children," said Malin, though she also loved her job and suspected she would never have been happy staying home full-time.

Feelings of guilt and self-recrimination could also be associated with caring for others' children. Elina had worked for a family where the mother had died and the father showed little concern for the children. When she left to move on in her own life she berated herself for letting them down, a sense that was brought home with painful clarity later when she visited the family and the youngest child asked, "Why did you leave me?"

As the primary parental caregivers, the women were not only subject to self-criticism, they were also the target of reproach. "I might get a tongue-lashing," said Linnea. "People would come up and say, 'Shouldn't that boy be wearing mittens? What kind of mother are you?'" It was pointless to explain that her psychologically disturbed son tore them off as soon as she put them on him. When she sought medical help she was told that she was to blame for his difficulties because she treated him inappropriately. It was years before the handicap was assigned a name: autism.

The women were also influenced by the knowledge and viewpoints of experts. Gertrud had found a childcare arrangement that worked well both for her and for the children. When she started studying child psychology and learned how vital a stay-at-home mother was, she was overcome by feelings of guilt. "I felt terrible deep inside, thinking I might have ruined something for my children." In retrospect she sometimes regretted having been so ambitious and focused on her job. Though she knew better and though the children also had a father, she came to believe the sole responsibility was hers, both for the children's welfare and for her own feelings of guilt.

Father-child relations

A couple of the women had also felt guilty about or had been blamed for the children's poor relationship with their father. That was Elina's experience. Periodically she took her daughter with her to visit her parents in Finland; at home she felt isolated, especially since her husband, a competitive skier, often chose to be away evenings and weekends. "Our daughter didn't really feel he was her father." Later, when the girl did not warm up to him, he blamed Elina's absences for causing the disconnect between them. "He didn't see that he himself could have stayed home more."

Several women were also continuously on their guard to fend off disagreements between fathers and children. Preventing arguments and expressing their own opinions were often difficult; the women felt caught in the middle. Sara still reproached herself for remaining silent. "Mostly I sat there quiet as a mouse, unfortunately. I should have put up a fuss." Elina never placed demands on her husband when her daughter was home for fear that he would then start ordering the girl around. At the dinner table she talked continuously to avert arguments. Worrying about "how it would go this evening" was constant, even when she was at work, and exhausted her. Consequently it was a big relief when her daughter grew up and left home.

A sense of accomplishment

The women also recalled ways in which they felt gratified by their mothering. "In our home, the kids don't have anything to complain about, and that makes me feel pretty good," said Estrid, thus making a direct connection between her own health and her role as a mother. That their children made it clear "they knew they were loved" helped the women accept their perceived shortcomings. Sara, who had felt "Inadequate almost all the time," eventually gained a different perspective and thought she had done the best she could. "Raising kids is an important contribution," said Signe, looking back on her life's work. Her children's testimony about how much she had meant to them also comforted her when she remembered the difficult years after her husband's untimely death, when money was tight. "It's a good thing you were the one who survived, they said. They knew they wouldn't have had a place to call home otherwise." On her own, she had managed to keep the family together, which none of the children thought their father could have done. She was also gratified by the emotional support she had given her brood. "I never left a child alone at bedtime – that's not on my conscience. I stroked their backs until they fell asleep."

The women had also received recognition for their engagement with their children. Signe could still call to mind the words of a teacher: "This is a mother who always puts her children first." Anna recalled that the physician at the children's clinic had praised her because her children were not overweight. "The others were clearly too fat. I was so proud." Despite all her domestic chores and work on the farm, she also felt she had done a good job of keeping an eye on the children and being available to them when they were small. "Sometimes they were in the fields, sometimes they were home. They pretty much took care of themselves. It's never been a problem for us."

At the time of the interviews the women's children and foster children were well into adulthood. That they had turned out well and found satisfaction at work and in their private lives gave the women a sense of security and reinforced their sense that they had done a good job as mothers. Several were particularly pleased that their children seemed to have better relationships with spouses and children than was the case in the parental generation. Sara observed with pleasure that her daughter had been able to implement a more equal division of household labor, while Gertrud was glad that her son had "learned to get by on his own."

Adult children and grandchildren

The women's involvement with their children continued after they had grown up. Those who became grandmothers took on new responsibilities, and caring for grandchildren gave some of them a chance to "make up for" a perceived neglect of their own children. Nearly everyone had been available to babysit; some were still doing so regularly. "Sometimes I wonder how they'd manage without me," said Linnea. Grandchildren also stayed overnight occasionally, and several women had provided daycare for varying lengths of time. Elna, who had to retire from her job for health reasons, had subsequently devoted virtually all her time to grandchildren, and later great-grandchildren. "It was thanks to me that my daughter could take a job – she had a babysitter." Helping out also had a positive effect on Elna herself. She could endure and sometimes even forget her physical symptoms and had more energy than she believed she would have had otherwise.

Geographical distance, illness, or lack of energy nevertheless limited the involvement of some women. This was the case for Sara, who "missed having someone to care for." Others found themselves too much in demand. Signe lived next door to one of her children and felt pressured. If there were difficulties with the grandchildren, she knew about them immediately: "Over time, I've become more sensitive to how the kids are doing. I can't do or say anything, but I recognize and register problems. Then I can't sleep." The women's own wellbeing was thus still dependent on the welfare of children and grandchildren.

Children of all ages were also considerate of their mothers. "The children spoil me to death," as Greta put it. Valborg described the same kind of concern: "My son comes over and washes the windows. He cares about his mother, you see." Adult children and their mothers might also do fun things together. Some had gone out dancing, many had traveled together, others were glad they could joke and be playful when they met. A number of the women felt they now were getting compensation for the years of hard work that raising children entailed.

Many were able to talk to their children about subjects they felt were important. Communication was often more open with daughters, but there were limits: those whose marriages had been troubled did not always want their children to know. Worries and illnesses were sometimes hidden so as "not to be a bother," and they did not want to become too dependent: "When I'm with the children everything is fine, but it's hard to accept that they can get tired of me," said Estrid.

Siblings, parents, and other relatives

Caregiving was sometimes reciprocal and sometimes more one-sided between the women and their parents and siblings. For some, a brother or sister had been especially important. "He understood without my saying anything – he could see..." said Elina of a younger brother. With regard to her unhappy marriage, she felt he was "the only person on earth" she could talk to. "My sister has been a rock, my strongest supporter," said Malin. When relationships were very close, concern for each other had been mutual.

For a couple of the women, however, taking care of a sibling had been a one-sided obligation. Elna "didn't have much choice" about helping her sister and her children; her choice of words suggests she was ambivalent about the task. "I was impatient and felt used, but she was sick, so there was nothing to be done about it." Elna also helped her brothers and their families, and when her parents were old and ill the caregiving responsibilities once again fell to her. Her four brothers "didn't have the emotional strength" and had "families of their own to consider." She herself was divorced, with children still living at home. None of the siblings ever acknowledged her caregiving efforts, but nieces and nephews later expressed their appreciation and affection.

Several women had cared for their parents for extended periods of time, an experience they looked back on with mixed feelings. They had felt needed, and in some instances had grown very close to their parents, but the burden of caregiving had often been overwhelming and impossible to avoid. Frida recalled that she had managed to care for both her mother and her invalid husband but had lost her voice. "For a long time I barely had the energy to speak." In contrast, Britt-

Marie, whose mother had died young, burst out, "If only I'd been able to fuss over my mother when I got on in years!" Living alone, with no siblings and no children of her own, she longed for a sense of connection. Earlier she had gained strength from caring for her father during his last illness. After his death she completely lost her bearings: "I didn't think I had any anchoring on earth and might just blow away. I gained a lot of weight, thinking that might hold me down."

Anna, the farmer's wife, found out that others considered it a given that she would be responsible for all caregiving in the home, even of her husband's parents. Since her mother-in-law had grown senile and was bedridden, this was a demanding task. It was also problematic when visiting in-laws tried to intervene without being willing to help. Anna thought the other women should have realized how overworked she was and shared the burden rather than criticizing. A happy memory was nevertheless that her mother-in-law intermittently showed appreciation for her efforts and that neighbors praised her devotion.

As mentioned previously, Blenda had assumed responsibility for the household, the farm, and her younger siblings when she was scarcely twenty. Ten years later, when one of her brothers got married, she was suddenly expected to vacate the home where she had grown up so that her sister-in-law, ten years younger, could take over as mistress of the house. Blenda had not been able to put aside anything to fall back on. She became physically ill and was overcome by feelings of inadequacy. "I was homeless and had no skills except housekeeping. It was terribly difficult and very frightening." Elna had also been pressured into leaving the family farm when her brothers and their wives asserted their rights of inheritance and domicile. Both Blenda and Elna learned that among siblings, equality and sharing did not always pertain. A contributing factor, both of them believed, was that without a husband they were viewed as lacking a family, despite the fact that both had children. Blenda was eventually able to return to her home district and was treated well by other relatives. "The family has been like a protective cloak," as she put it.

For Elina from Finland, contact with relatives in the homeland meant a connection to her childhood, her own history, and her native language. Along with the family's characteristic sense of humor, this was what she looked forward to on her yearly visits to the village she came from.

Several women who had established good relations with their husbands' families soon discovered that it was they, not their husbands, who were expected to stay in touch. "That it would turn out this way wasn't something you expected when you got married," said Sara, noting that she was the one who purchased all the presents and planned all the parties, even for her husband's family.

5

Running a Household

Social and political reform

As previously noted, the period during which the women in this study were running a household coincided with the establishment and growth of the Swedish welfare state or "People's Home." The concept encompasses a lengthy period of social-democratic political rule extending from 1932 until 2006, with brief interruptions during the 1970s and '80s.[16]

Above all, the focus was on improving the wretched living conditions and poor health of the working class. With an increased awareness of the impact of housing on health issues, the goal was that all members of society would have access to running water and indoor plumbing. Beginning in the 1930s, the norm in newly constructed buildings, often municipally run, was a bathroom in each apartment. In an effort to combat overcrowded conditions, rooms were larger than previously and let in more light. By today's standards, however, space remained limited. For instance, in Stockholm, the Swedish capital, the requirement for renting a small apartment (two rooms, kitchen and bath) in one of the so-called "large family buildings"[17] was that the family included at least three children. Well into the 1950s, the most common family dwelling in Stockholm consisted of a single room with kitchen, and far from everyone had access to comfortable living conditions. In rural areas, too, housing was crowded, and modern conveniences were often lacking. Sparsely populated parts of the country did not have electricity until the middle of the century.

---

16 Between 2006 and 2014, Sweden was ruled by a coalition of bourgeois (non-socialist) parties. The state-supported system of security embracing everyone irrespective of class, described earlier in this book, was partially dismantled under the bourgeois government.
17 In 1935, the Swedish parliament decreed that apartment buildings should be built specifically for low-income families with many children, whose current living conditions were defined as overcrowded.

In other words, at mid-century many people did not have housing that met modern standards. Household work was demanding and carried out almost exclusively by women. In an attempt to raise the status of housework and caregiving, a state institute for research on work within the home was established.[18] Various tasks performed in the home were studied in detail; experts provided advice and suggested more effective techniques. Though the goal of improving the status of housework was never achieved, the activities of the institute led to better kitchen and household equipment to help make housework easier. Another attempt to upgrade the status of work within the home was to calculate its economic value for the nation. This effort also failed. Down to the present, work for pay has retained higher social status than the unpaid work of running a household.

All the women in our study had primary responsibility for their households, but initially with widely varying skills. "I was an idiot when it came to housekeeping," said Sara. She and others, however, acquired the skills needed, if not before, then after having children. In this chapter they describe their working conditions and what running a household entailed.

Money and control

The women's economic situation had a major influence on the time and effort devoted to housework. Lack of money made everyday life more difficult. This was especially problematic for the two women who were raising children alone. Both worked full-time at low-paying jobs. "We didn't have enough money for anything – food, clothes, you name it," said Elna. "We could barely afford a dish cloth. I was always counting in my head to be sure we could cover expenses," said Blenda.

Several of the married women also described financial difficulties. Often their own needs came last; they might freeze or go hungry because their children, and their husbands, were given first priority. External circumstances also affected economic matters. In Hungary, Irina's first home as a newlywed was completely destroyed during the war. By the time she and her husband had built up a new one, the political situation had become so intolerable that they were forced to flee and came to Sweden. "The worst of it at first was being poor," Irina said. "We had only a few small suitcases with us when we arrived." It was particularly difficult to outfit the children for school. No government

---

18 Hemmets forskningsinstitut (Home Research Institute, 1944); later Statens Konsumentverk (Swedish Consumer Agency).

assistance was available; they had to borrow money to buy furniture and household items. For Irina and her family, the skills and behavior patterns acquired during years of enforced thrift remained in place even after their economic situation had improved.

Her husband's stinginess meant that Greta seldom had enough money, even to cover official responsibilities connected with the rectory. She was forced to beg him for everything except money for food. "It was almost like being declared incompetent." What money there was he reserved for himself, for instance to buy a new car, a film camera or other "unnecessary" items. To have money of her own, Greta picked berries in the forest and sold them. She also sewed most of her own clothes and those of the children. As soon as she could, she returned to her previous job as a midwife and district nurse.

As we have already seen, several other women were also dependent on their husbands to cover household expenses. Valborg kept a close watch trying to prevent her husband from spending money on alcohol; Karin never got the car that would have lightened her workload. Although Anna's marriage was harmonious, it was nevertheless her husband who had the last word on financial matters.

Britt-Marie, who had ruled out marriage because she did not think she could handle waiting on a husband, never learned anything about housekeeping. Since she lived alone, she felt she did not need to. "I've never had a household," she said, expressing the prevailing view that a household of one was not a "real" household. As a working woman, she could afford to buy prepared food, and she paid others to do cleaning and laundry.

The work environment

The time and energy needed for housework was determined not only by financial circumstances and family size, but also by the layout and comfort level of the dwelling. Living conditions for many participants in the study were crowded and many did not have modern conveniences. Malin, an executive secretary, lived in two rooms and a kitchen with six other people, including a maid and her mother-in-law. Much time and effort was required to set up beds for everyone in the evening and put everything away again in the morning.

Several women in rural areas lived in houses without running water during the most demanding years of their work lives. They fetched water from wells or lakes, carried in wood to light the stove that provided heat and a cooking surface, and had no indoor toilet. Signe's small house was not updated until the 1960s, when most of her brood had left home. City apartments could also be substandard. Klary, a factory worker in a large metropolitan area, did not have hot water and central heating until the mid-1970s, only a cold-water faucet in the kitchen. She did not dare leave the kerosene heaters on during the day. "It was cold when you got home from work," she said.

In the 1930s and '40s, housekeeping demands might also differ between married women and those who were single. As previously mentioned, the unmarried schoolteacher Marta was assumed not to need modern conveniences. She was housed on the second floor of the school building. Water and wood had to be carried up the stairs and garbage carried down. In the winter it was icy and slippery. She recalled her anger after falling, garbage pail in hand, and injuring herself.

The external environment and the distance to stores, laundry facilities, and other services were also factors affecting the workload. The teacher Sara moved with her family to a more elegant apartment when her husband was promoted. Circumstances changed, but hardly for the better from Sara's perspective: it was a longer walk to the store and the new apartment was more difficult to clean. Karin, the principal's wife in charge of a large house, also lived far from stores and other services.

A number of women living in houses found that tasks usually performed by men often fell to them, a development they had not foreseen when they married. Greta, for instance, had not expected to be shoveling snow from the rectory driveway. It was heavy work and could take several hours. Elina, who suffered from a painful hip ailment, also felt it necessary to take on snow-shoveling chores. "Sometimes I felt sad when I came home and saw snow on the bridge and he was already inside." Sara described climbing up on the roof of the house several times to do repairs. "I did it even though I really didn't have the strength," she said. Estrid, in contrast, had felt strong and enjoyed heavy labor. She helped drill the foundation for the family's house, chopped wood, and did most of the gardening.

Even if it was substandard, a home of one's own was often valued very highly. Among the positive aspects of living in a house was proximity to nature: perhaps a sunny step to sit on, a yard to enjoy. Signe remembered her pleasure returning home after visiting others who might be better off. She would think, "I do have a nice home – flowers, dishes, rag rugs. I'm comfortable here."

Working together with other women was important for many. In rural areas women might do the baking with neighbors and relatives and help each other with laundry and other heavy tasks. Being able to see and talk to other adults was a significant positive factor in the work environment. In cities, women working at home also saw to it that they met during "work hours." "We formed our own work group," as Karin saw it. "We helped each other with the children and met in each other's homes." Sewing bees in particular could function as a kind of common workplace for handiwork as well as a discussion forum. If meetings were in the evening women with salaried jobs could also participate. Interacting with other housewives nevertheless did not appeal to everyone. Linnea, the physician, felt out of place in this context and always longed to return to her profession.

Recognition for the work they did was also an issue connected with the quality of the work environment. Many felt their husbands were completely unaware of their workload and consequently neither understood its scope nor respected their efforts. Even women who described their marriages as good felt let down. "They don't see everything you do unless you point it out, just think it happens on its own," was Signe's representative comment. She had occasionally thought that if she were to die, her husband would marry "anyone at all in a skirt" to have someone to take care of hearth and home.

Cleaning

Many women commented on what a heavy burden cleaning could be. "You lay there scrubbing until your arms were out of joint," recalled Elna, who lived with her parents and children in a large house without modern updates. Others described mopping, scouring, dusting off, airing out, carrying out rugs, changing bedding, wiping out cabinets, and washing windows, in a constant stream of tasks. Many noted repeatedly that cleaning was work that never ended. "There was sand everywhere. You cleaned and cleaned, and it was the same the next day," said Elina. She despised cleaning, but wanted their house to be welcoming to her daughter and her friends.

In addition to daily cleaning, there were weekly and seasonal cleaning chores. In rural households these included regular cleaning of barns, out-buildings, and baking huts. "In the spring everything had to be scrubbed down, from the cellar to the roof of the storage shed," said Anna. Women with paying jobs often did the cleaning on weekends. Those who were employed as cleaners experienced this as especially dreary and exhausting. There was nevertheless one advantage to housework: "You could start and stop when you yourself chose to."

The women also described what happened with the cleaning when they were ill for an extended period. Frida found it painful to watch the chores "piling up" without having the energy to take anything on. At the time of the interviews, some women were ailing or disabled and needed help with cleaning, but they nevertheless continued doing as much as they could. Marta, the artist who had gone blind, mopped the floors herself, which made her feel they were truly clean even though she could not see them. Her greatest concern was that everything took so much longer – cooking, cleaning, laundry. Gertrud found it difficult to "watch everything go to wrack and ruin." She did have help, but not for everything she considered necessary.

Laundry

Doing the family laundry was also a heavy chore, especially for women with large families and no running water. In the summer, Signe washed all her children's clothes in the sea; in the winter she had to manage in the kitchen. She used the children's bathwater and then dried the laundry on clotheslines above the stove. Cloth diapers were also washed by hand; disposable ones did not yet exist. To reach an actual laundry facility she had to go to the mainland by boat or walk across the ice. She took sheets and other large items there, returning the next day to put them through the mangle. Though she longed for a laundry room of her own, she did not get one while her children were young. Her husband's attitude was the determining factor: he was convinced that since she "seemed to enjoy doing laundry so much" she would then spend all her time in the laundry room. The comment is perhaps best understood as evidence of an inability to recognize just how arduous and time-consuming a chore the laundry was.

For a long time, laundry facilities in cities were not up-to-date, either, and might be far away. Estrid described "hauling big loads of laundry quite a distance"; Valborg "dragged the laundry down the street." "Small stuff," that is, underwear and children's clothing, was often washed by hand at home. A separate chore was taking care of laundry connected to the women's menstrual periods. Before the existence of disposable pads and tampons, women used cloth pads that had to be washed. Bloodstained clothing and bed linens also led to additional laundry, especially for women with heavy periods.

How the women experienced their work also depended on who it was performed for. This came out in connection with ironing. Elna recalled her irritation at having to iron her brothers' shirts, comparing this to the pleasure of ironing baby clothing: "That was delightful – it smelled like baby."

When washing machines arrived in the 1950s, they required much more attention and manual work than present-day machines. Even so, they eased the everyday burden considerably. "It was almost a bigger event than getting running water," said Anna, who prior to this had done the family laundry in a cauldron in the barn. When we interviewed the women, laundry remained a heavy daily chore for those providing home care to ill husbands. "I'm worn out – my legs, my whole body is done in," said Valborg, whose husband was bedridden and incontinent. Though she was old and tired herself, every morning she had to carry sheets and covers to the laundry room and back.

Food preparation

Regardless of training and interest, all the women had been responsible for cooking for their families. For those whose husbands and children ate all meals at home, this meant preparing and serving many meals each day. Farmers' wives, who often had large households, were particularly burdened. "Breakfast at nine, fish, potatoes, porridge. Dinner at one. Porridge in the evening. In between, coffee and a snack," recalled Anna. City-dwelling Estrid prepared five lunch boxes before leaving for work each day: three for sons who lived at home, one for her husband, and one for herself.

Planning the meals was considered a big job in itself – it was important to think everything through carefully. Signe was always worried there would not be enough for everyone. The food also needed to be healthy and varied. "Worry about what to make – I've always done that, to avoid always having the same thing," said Gertrud. Many women, especially those with large families, also baked all their own bread.

Women with paying jobs described the daily stress connected with putting food on the table. "I was in a rush to get home in the evening. They were hungry then, of course, and I had to buy food along the way," said Malin. Family finances determined what the women could buy and where they could buy it. Those with little money spent a great deal of time comparing prices at different shops, and some women could rarely afford vegetables.

Bringing food and other goods back home was also a demanding task that without exception was performed by the women. Linnea "walked and carried things" while her husband used the car for his own purposes. Estrid was afraid her bicycle, weighed down with heavy bags of food, would tip over. A couple of the women blamed pain in shoulders, neck, and arms on their many years of "hauling things home."

Far from everyone was good at or enjoyed cooking. "For me it has just been a boring obligation," said Malin. Greta always had "a complex" about her cooking. Sara thought "cooking is just something you have to do." Valborg used the expression "long vacation" about a period of hospitalization when meals were served to her. Blenda, in contrast, was among those who enjoyed cooking, but for a long time she could not afford what she wanted. Still, her knowledge of food meant she was able to prepare good, nutritious meals at little cost.

Using what the household produced was an important and sometimes necessary part of food preparation for some. Anna was responsible for turning products from animals and the vegetable garden into ready meals. "Nothing could go to waste. We slaughtered pigs, salted and smoked the pork and put it in the ice shed. In those days we didn't have a freezer." Karin had a garden that necessitated a great deal of work. A number of women also mentioned what a chore it was to go out in the woods each fall and pick enough berries of various kinds to last through the winter.

During the war years (1939-1945) special conditions pertained, including shortages and rationing of food items, shoes, and clothing, that presented increased challenges to the skills and creativity of housewives. In Hungary, Irina's mother's garden saved the family from starving. Even in Sweden, allotments to each individual in a household were limited. Estrid mentioned how valuable it was that her husband could bring back meat from the area where he was stationed. For a long time, Klary saved her vouchers for coffee, meat, eggs, and butter so she could arrange a party when she got married.

Clothes and other textiles

Providing the family with clean and mended clothes occupied much of the women's time. Like food preparation, this was an area in which the women's skills and ingenuity could have a significant effect on the family's finances. Sewing and altering clothes was frequently necessary to stay within budget. This applied to the unmarried mothers, to those with large families, and also to the minister's wife Greta, who got no money for clothes from her husband.

It was important that the children looked "nice and properly dressed." If there was only one change of clothing neither laundry nor mending could be postponed – work might have to be done in the evenings and on weekends. "You had to sit there in the evening when they'd fallen asleep and early in the morning before they woke up, sewing, patching, mending stockings," said Signe. Some of the women were well enough off to "buy ready-made," but even they thought taking care of children's clothing took a lot of time. It was hard to find suitable items in stores, and even nice clothes tore and needed to be mended. Karin thought she always had the sewing machine out. Sara, who was pressed for time and did not like sewing, pasted patches onto the legs of the children's pants with textile glue. In old age some women were still mending and patching things, even though it might not be necessary. "I admit it. I still mend stockings for my husband and myself. You save quite a bit," said Irina.

Sewing, as well as knitting, crocheting, and weaving, was thus in many instances necessary to keep the family in clothes. At the same time the women longed to "make something beautiful," but often there was only time for essentials. "Crocheting pretty things was a luxury we couldn't afford," said Signe – but later it came out that she had, in fact, crocheted lace borders on her daughters' undergarments. Other textiles – bedclothes, tablecloths, and curtains – also required time-consuming care and were intended to be beautiful and a source of pride. "Everything in the linen cabinet was supposed to be mangled smooth and flat, with curled ribbons on the pillowcases."

Later, when the children had left home, embroidery, handiwork, and weaving might be for pleasure rather than out of necessity. A number of women found satisfaction in "making something to pass on." Handiwork could also be restful and create the sense of being at peace, of having "a space of one's own within the room." The work satisfied the requirement of "always having busy hands," but made it possible for thoughts to wander freely. For Elina, handiwork was a way of keeping at bay the frightening images that often filled the television screen, reminding her of the war she herself had experienced.

Guests

The women described what it was like to organize parties on major holidays or other festive occasions. Even those who did not like household work enjoyed planning a party now and then. But inviting people over was not always a simple matter. The expectation that food and baked goods had to be "elegant" might be an impediment, and sometimes women had neither the time nor the energy. Some also lacked the financial resources. "It ended up that I almost didn't dare have guests," said Malin, afraid of not being able to live up to expectations. "It wasn't just the food part. There was supposed to be fruit and something to drink and flowers on the table." Frida would also have preferred less fuss connected with getting together. "It would have been nice to have friends you could drop in on, just like that," she said.

The Christmas holiday required an extra effort. The teacher, Sara, described a high stress level, both at home and in school. Arranging big Christmas gatherings under these circumstances pressed her to the limit but also brought pleasure and gratification. Others described what transpired when adult children came home to visit. Signe, with her ten children, might have twenty people sleeping at her house. At the time of the interviews she no longer had space for her loom. Beds for visiting children and grandchildren occupied the place where it once had stood.

Uninvited guests might also turn up, especially if the women had remained in their home districts. Relatives returning home might appear at any time and expect to be fed and housed. "They did help out, but…" said Elna, who worked full-time outside the home but felt she had to take on most of the burden herself when kinfolk came to visit.

In retrospect

Among the women who worked solely within the home, several had originally envisioned something else. Signe had dreamed of working in a shop, but had neither time nor energy enough for that. In retrospect she felt she had had no choice and that it was a significant accomplishment to bring up ten children.

Taking care of a home in accordance with one's own criteria, and those of others, was important. During the so-called housewife period of the 1930s, '40s, and '50s, there was a great deal of expert advice, not only on childcare but also on housekeeping. Whether working within or outside the home, women wanted to live up to these standards.

Over time, several women had attempted to lower their own expectations for a properly run household with regard to cooking, cleaning, and clothing the family. This was not always easy, as Sara expressed with the words, "I've tried just letting things go, but can't stand looking at the mess – you're the one who suffers the most." Or as Gertrud put it, "Now he thinks I shouldn't do thus and such. But then what am I supposed to do if it doesn't get done?"

Karin knew she had been a good housewife, taking care of her family and helping her husband in his work. She had chosen not to have either a nanny or a maid, as was customary in her social position. Her decision to stop working as a dental hygienist and stay at home was in keeping with the prevailing social norms and political ideology of the time. In the 1950s and '60s, toward the end of the most demanding years of her work life, social values shifted as more and more women looked for employment outside the home. Karin's decades of labor were now seen as a "life of luxury" and housewives were considered "spoiled." More than once she overheard comments like "She's just a stay-at-home wife" or "What does she do all day?" – making her occasionally question the value of her skills and what she had actually accomplished during all those years.

6

In the Work Force

Women and the labor market

When study participants entered the labor market in the 1930s and '40s, it was strictly segregated by gender in accordance with traditional perceptions of the type of work men and women were best suited for. Men held the vast majority of higher positions, though women were not unheard of. The first woman member of parliament took her seat in the 1920s, the first woman holding a professorship of medicine in the 1930s, and the first cabinet minister in the 1940s.

For unmarried middle-class women, jobs in education (teaching) and the caring professions (nursing and midwifery) were considered most appropriate. A low-level position in business and administration, as a post office clerk, telegraph operator, or office worker, might also be a possibility. Working-class women almost always ended up in physically demanding jobs, in kitchens and households of the well-to-do, as shop attendants, in industry, and in agriculture. Since apprenticeships and other training positions were reserved for men, women were blocked from better-paying jobs. That was also the outcome of the ban on night labor for female factory workers that was put in place early in the century, though it was motivated by concern for the health of women and unborn children. The ban was lifted only in the 1960s. A comparable prohibition on working the night shift in hospitals and care facilities was never considered.

Married women's right to be in the work force remained a topic of intense debate. In the 1930s it was by no means a given that women could retain their jobs after marrying or becoming pregnant. The political ideal of the housewife and the goal that "one salary should support an entire family" prevailed throughout society. Before her marriage, one woman in the study, the secretary Malin, had gone to her boss and expressed the desire to keep her job. That her request was granted may be connected to a wider discussion of women's rights in the labor market, promoted by a special government committee, and by an awareness that the approaching war in Europe would call for more women in the work force. Shortly thereafter, in 1939, parliament voted to prohibit the dismissal of women when their marital status changed or they had children.

Despite legislative changes, the social norm of the housewife remained in place for the next several decades. The ideal notwithstanding, a single income – the husband's – was not always enough to support a family. For that reason many women took on work outside the home, often work that fell outside the regular labor market. They might do housecleaning, deliver newspapers, pick berries, or work in a shop and were paid by the hour, with little job security and irregular working hours. This type of arrangement gave employers access to a work force that was low-cost and flexible, and with luck the women could adjust the workload and schedule to fit in with the needs of their families. Since couples were taxed as a unit, this type of untaxed work meant more money in the pocket, at least for the time being, than employment in the regular labor market. It did not, however, provide social benefits such as sick leave compensation, disability payments, or a pension based on salaried earnings.

Women married to farmers were not registered as members of the work force until the mid-1960s and it took another decade before their labor qualified them for a pension beyond the base level paid to everyone. When women employed outside the regular labor market and farm wives are included in the statistics for working women, the picture differs significantly from what is usually presented. The official number of housewives – 1.5 million in a population of slightly less than 8 million – is misleading, as is the supposed fall-off in the number of working women during the 1940s and '50s. In reality, women have always had a high level of participation in the labor market, but their contribution has not always been included in the statistics.

All the women in this study had, at some point in their lives, worked for pay, whether in the regular work force or outside it. For many, including those who were married, work had been an economic necessity. Nearly half the women had always had salaried employment except during brief periods after childbirth. Among those who stopped working when they got married, several returned to their professions when the children were older.

A significant subset of the women lacked a formal education past primary school, and some had begun their adult working lives while still in their early teens. Women who grew up in farming families helped out at home or worked on other farms, in the household or the barn. Those who came from working-class families, whether rural or urban, were also likely to find work in others' homes, as maids or nannies. Some later worked on large estates, in shops, at laundries or as cleaners, or found factory jobs. The informal training in housekeeping and caregiving that they had received while growing up, and later by working in their own homes, often made it easy for them to take on a broad range of tasks in the work force. This applied, for instance, to Blenda, who toward the end of her working life provided home services for the elderly, but had previously worked on a farm, as a maid, in industrial kitchens, and as a waitress.

Among the women with a secondary education, there were one office worker, two nurses, one dental hygienist, one primary school teacher (later an artist), one telegraph operator, one engineer, and one hairdresser. Two women earned a university degree; one became a secondary school teacher, the other a physician.

During the economic crisis of the 1930s unemployment was high, and women, especially those with little formal education, had to take whatever work they could find, often with little job security. Klary, who worked in a shoe factory, related that when the raw materials ran out, she and the other women had to sit waiting for a new shipment. They received no pay during this time, since wages were entirely dependent on the piecework rate. In the summers, when the factory closed, they were unemployed; there was no paid vacation.[19] Estrid's situation was equally insecure. She had grown up among indentured farm workers but moved to an urban area in search of a job. When she eventually managed to find one in a hotel kitchen it was through personal contacts.

Work prospects grew better during World War II. Though Sweden was not a combatant, the country was isolated from the outside world and everyday life was affected in many ways. For both men and women, unemployment disappeared. Women were now needed in what had previously been strictly male sectors to replace men who had been drafted for military service. Altered circumstances during these years of "preparedness" also called for new products and services. The shoe factory where Klary worked began producing gas masks; there were no work interruptions, and pay improved. Elna, who was in "desperate need of an income" after a divorce, recalled that during this period it was easy to find all kinds of work and possible to hold several jobs simultaneously. After the war ended, women were once again denied access to many types of salaried work to make place for men returning

---

19 In 1938 parliament passed a law establishing the right to two weeks of paid vacation each year. The length has gradually been extended and is currently five weeks, often longer for those in higher positions.

from military service. When women took over men's work, however, the effects were not always positive. On farms, the burden of labor might become overwhelming. In Finland, Elina, still a teenager, had seriously injured herself working in the fields and in the forest, taking over for brothers killed in battle.

During the economic expansion of the 1950s there was once again a demand for women in the labor market. In cities many women found jobs in industry. Estrid related that "at that time there was also a shortage of people who knew how to clean" – an employer had "begged" for her services. Women who were middle-aged or older were also needed, not least in the rapidly growing public sector. Housewives and women whose previous work had been outside the regular labor market could often step directly into such positions. To make it more lucrative for married women to work for pay, joint taxation for couples was eliminated in 1971. Part-time work was nevertheless common, especially among older women, and in that generation a woman's income was still seen primarily as a complement to her husband's and not intended to make her self-supporting.

In rural areas there might still be few jobs for women. Elna noted that men quit their jobs at the local textile factory because they were so poorly paid. They could find other jobs, while the women were forced to stay, having no other options. Elina, who moved to Sweden at this time, found her options limited because she did not know the language. "All the Finnish women were cleaning ladies," she said.

As noted, the lack of public childcare facilities was a major problem at the beginning of this period. Only during the 1970s, after insistent pressure from various women's organizations, did an extensive expansion of daycare centers begin. Along with successive improvements in parental leave policy, this gradually made it less difficult for women to combine childbearing, motherhood, and work for pay. Debate about men's increased involvement in housework and childcare also intensified. In practice, women still bore primary responsibility for work in the home.

Gender-based salaries

During the entire twentieth century, wages in female-dominated fields such as nursing and the service professions were lower than those in occupations dominated by men, a situation that continues today. The sociologist Alva Myrdal commented in the 1930s that it had become a tradition to equate low-paying work with women's work. "This always functions reciprocally," she wrote. "Work that is underpaid will be seen as appropriate for women, while work that is seen as especially appropriate for women will be underpaid" (Myrdal 1938: 32-33). Even when men and women held the same job, employers had the legal right until the 1960s to pay women less. The justification was that men, but not women, were responsible for supporting their families, a claim that did not always correspond with reality. Elna, working at a textile factory, earned less than the men, including the apprentices she herself trained. She brought up the unfair pay scale in the union she helped establish but never got a response. Klary, who after her piecework job at the shoe factory found work with an hourly wage at a cable factory, related, "A fellow who put up the cable lines was paid quite a bit more. My job was more strenuous, but brought in less." Klary's husband, who had a similar job in the same factory, also received higher wages although she had worked there longer. She felt the wage scale was unfair but had not complained. "You were used to it, saw it as something natural since it was that way for everyone." In contrast, the secondary school teacher earned the same salary and received the same pension as her husband. "The only difference was that I had a second job once I came home," Sara said.

As noted previously, women's wages at mid-century were still so low that unmarried women, even those without children, had difficulty getting by and could not afford housing of their own. One way to solve the housing problem was to take a position as a maid, like Blenda in our study, or as a nanny. Both were common job categories for women, though wages were extremely low and work hours unregulated. In the 1940s a law was passed that set a limit – though a high one – on work hours for maids, but not for those minding children. Later, when Blenda worked in an industrial kitchen, she was still very poorly paid. Someone who had seen her paycheck called it "starvation wages." She nevertheless refused to join the union, since she did not want her meager salary to go toward further raising the pay of the men; she had no expectation that they would help her. Even nurses, despite years of training and positions with great responsibility, could scarcely live on their income.

Edit, married to a grocer, had taken almost no pay for her work in the shop. Since couples were taxed jointly, there was no advantage to the family if she had an income, but as a consequence she ended up with a very small pension. Women married to farmers had no taxable income at all; though they played a major role in farm production, they were considered housewives. This was the situation for Anna, who stated that she "didn't earn anything" and did not see herself as being in the work force, despite the fact that the milking and her work in the store brought in much of the family's cash.

Knowing one's place

The women described being assigned less attractive jobs than their male co-workers and having fewer possibilities for advancement. Unlike the men, neither Klary nor Elna, both working strenuous factory jobs, could advance to foreman. Though all cleaners, like Valborg, were female, the boss was a man. "Cleaners were worth less than nothing," she said, referring to the offensive treatment they endured from him. He was stingy even when it came to the essential tools of the trade, cleaning rags: "There had to be a big hole before you got a new one." The women nevertheless banded together among themselves, drawing straws to determine who would take the most demanding tasks. The telegraph operator Britt-Marie likewise had only female colleagues but male bosses, who lacked the education and language training the profession required but were paid more.

The hierarchy became clear to Greta, the district nurse, when she worked with physicians who outranked her but whom she nevertheless needed to train. The physician Linnea saw the female staff favor her male colleagues and "put them on a pedestal." She felt that she herself was often criticized and called into question because she was a woman. "It's as if you're always reminded to know your place." Vera, the engineer, who worked for many years at a tannery where virtually all employees were men, often felt cut off from others as the lone woman in a high position.

In contrast, as an artist Marta did not think there was gender discrimination in her profession, but added that she had always stayed in the background rather than trying to attract attention, as many of her male compatriots did. Malin, the executive secretary, also felt that women could achieve "some sort of equality" with regard to work and career. She herself advanced to a middle-level position with considerable autonomy, though she continued to provide personal services to her male bosses, something she saw as "natural."

Sexual harassment

For some of the women, sexual attraction and erotic currents were an enjoyable part of the job. Blenda, working in an industrial kitchen, mentioned, for instance, "flirting among the cases of beer." On the other hand, she and about half of the other women also described unwanted sexual comments or advances. In Elna's case, it was the boss at the textile factory who came down into the cellar and "wanted to touch my breasts, put his arm around me." She had rebuffed him and threatened to tell others if he continued. With Estrid, who cleaned at construction sites, it was one of the workers who "made brazen comments." For both these women, the incidents were sporadic. Others had been harassed over an extended period, in particular those working in kitchens and as cleaners. "The worst part was going down to the fellows in the cellar," said Blenda, who went through the building with a coffee wagon. "They were incredibly crude, really off-putting. They pinched me and discovered I was ticklish. I was scared to death to go down there." Elina connected the sexual comments she encountered with her low position in the pecking order. "They said things they could only say to a cleaner." A male co-worker had also talked about "waiting for me on the way home," a threat that made her choose an alternative route. "I was frightened when we had the same evening shift," she said. Vera, the engineer, was also subjected to sexual advances from a co-worker. "For protection, I asked one of the foremen to sit next to me," she recalled.

Women working in the healthcare system had likewise experienced sexual harassment. While still a nursing student, Gertrud had been badgered by a patient, but had never dared tell anyone. Linnea, the physician, described "always having to be on guard against inappropriate advances" from colleagues. Frida had been groped by a doctor while riding the elevator. Later, discovering that a male physician was making sexual advances to female patients, she had protected them by staying in the room. "My being there kept him from doing anything with them," she said. She also made an effort to find remote and private examining rooms for women undergoing intimate procedures, a practice that was not always a given at the time.

Listening and being supportive

Women working in the healthcare system described the unspoken expectation that they would listen to and be supportive of those they were caring for. This affected the way they approached their jobs and was an unacknowledged component of the workload. Linnea, who as a gynecologist early in her professional life had the confidence of her patients, and knew she was as important to female patients as a middle-aged psychiatrist. She also believed she had a different perspective on their psychological problems than the male staff. "When the women came back from home visits the staff asked their *husbands* how things had gone. To me the women would confide that they were living in the worst marriage on earth." Patients of Greta, the district nurse, sometimes turned to her rather than the male physician. "They didn't think he'd be able to provide much actual help." Greta also was "on call" for women before women's crisis centers existed, which meant long work days and frequent overtime. "I knew some of them needed to come and talk, which had to be in the afternoon, after regular hours. I could offer support, maybe help them take the necessary steps, say 'You can't go on this way.'" Listening to others was also a major part of Greta's role as a minister's wife. Few were aware of her own difficult personal situation.

Close relationships with patients and sensitivity to their situations often made it difficult to set limits on involvement. Anxiety and guilt feelings were the result if they felt they did not measure up. When Linnea suffered from chronic fatigue, a painful aspect of her illness was the inability to empathize with her patients, the core of her work as a psychiatrist. Frida described "not being able to let go" of the patients when the work day was over. Sometimes the women were caught between the expectations of their superiors and the needs of the patients. "The chief surgeon had a way of showing you who was in charge," said the nurse Gertrud, recalling her role as mediator between him on the one hand and the rest of the staff and the patients on the other. She still had strong feelings of guilt about one occasion when she felt she had let someone down. A female patient had filed a complaint against the surgeon. Though Gertrud wanted to offer her full support, she could not bring herself to criticize her boss so openly.

In other professions as well, caring for others was part of the daily routine. As a grade school teacher, Marta was constantly aware of the children's needs. She might bring those who were hungry or sick upstairs to her apartment, where she could provide a wood-burning stove for warmth, a listening ear, and if needed, food. For Edit in the grocery shop, the joys and sorrows of the customers were part of the job. "Customers wanted someone to confide in," she said. The engineer Vera also described listening to confidential matters while at work. Both her bosses and her co-workers, all men, came to her with their troubles.

Time pressure

Female healthcare workers often felt they did not have enough time. Linnea recalled her first day on the job as a psychiatrist. "I started on a Monday. A new patient was scheduled every half hour. There were medical records piled this high. I hadn't met a single patient yet and read through the records until my eyes fell out. Almost all the patients were psychotic." Concerning the work situation as it later evolved, she said, "It seemed to me I had an absurd amount to do. I'm not sure how many patients were on the ward, maybe thirty, and far more than that on the floor for chronic patients. What kind of care is that? But since I'm quite ambitious, goodness how hard I worked!"

As a nurse, Frida recalled a steady stream of tasks to perform. "It was impossible to say you hadn't been able to get to something," she said. There was no time for a proper food break. Workweeks were long, with evening shifts and frequent night duty. In addition it was essential to remember everything and never make a mistake. "God save the person who didn't do a good job. You were expected to handle everything, and you never knew what was coming."

The lower a woman's position in the hierarchy, the less control she had over work hours. Valborg described assignments that were impossible to complete during regular hours, forcing all the cleaners to work overtime. In industry, piecework was the rule. For Elna at the textile factory, "Everything was supposed to go so fast. Two fifteen-minute breaks a day. We ate standing up most of the time, and there was barely time to go to the toilet." Overtime brought no extra pay but was required for the good of the firm. For Blenda, in the industrial kitchen, the pace was also "as fast as can be." There were "big barrels of herring that had to be cleaned, with bones that cut your fingers." Women in office jobs might also feel closely monitored. Britt-Marie, the telegraph operator, said, "I've always felt I'm under observation. At my level, you always had to work constantly, no chance of sitting there twiddling your thumbs."

Vera, the engineer, was "always on the go" and felt that having many irons in the fire was good for her. Unlike many of the other women, she was largely free to set her own work schedule. "I could take two hours for lunch if I wanted without asking anyone." Instead she often stayed late in the evening; work hours were flexible. The job was stimulating and others relied on her. "I could take charge and show initiative," she said. This was also true for Malin, who often stayed late at the office to clear off her desk. At the grocery shop, Edit described early mornings, late evenings, and extra work before weekends and holidays. "When you have your own shop you can't count the hours – there was no way to limit them," she said. Marta, the artist, also noted that practicing her craft occupied essentially every waking moment. Her best work time was late in the evening and at night, "since that's when it's calm and quiet, no phone calls, no interruptions."

Monotonous and strenuous work

The perception of women as patient and precise meant that they were considered particularly suitable for simple, repetitive tasks, both in industry and in the office. Klary described her first job: "At the shoe factory the work was tedious, the same thing over and over. I sewed the heels together, and that was the only thing I did." Her subsequent job at the cable factory was more varied, but also more strenuous. "There were enormous spools of wire the cables ran on that had to be mounted in the machines. It was heavy work, but you figured it out, used your knee to push." She went on, "Of course the men helped me if I asked, but you wanted to be capable of doing everything yourself." Being capable nevertheless had its price. "That comes later, of course," she said, referring to the chronic back problems she had had ever since.

Elna, who was physically small, related that male co-workers in the textile factory had less strenuous and more varied assignments than she. "Washing and dyeing were reserved for men – I don't know why. Spinning was harder on you." It was only in retrospect that she realized just how taxing it had been. "You had to lift nearly your own weight," she said.

Estrid's workday at a construction site began with removing material the workers had left behind, much of it heavy: wooden planks, cement, and so on. Valborg and other cleaning women had to carry heavy pails of water up many flights of stairs: "It was awful to carry so much up those stairs. It was a dog's life." Blenda, the kitchen worker, likewise described a great deal of heavy lifting. "Huge kettles for making pea soup that you cranked up. They were bigger than this table and could hold a hundred liters." There were also "huge potato pots," 50 liters of potatoes that had to be lifted to pour the water off. Worst of all was the "coffee wagon that weighed a ton" that was maneuvered into and out of elevators and between floors.

Unsatisfactory work environments and monotonous assignments were also common in other occupations. The office of Greta, the district nurse, was a windowless cellar room impossible to air out. By afternoon, after working there all day, she was often on the verge of fainting from the heat and lack of oxygen. Only when a physician reacted did things improve. It also took six years of "nagging" to get a typewriter, by which time extensive note-taking by hand had led to an inflammation of the wrist. When Britt-Marie's job as a telegraph operator became obsolete she was relegated to less qualified work recording statistics. "Endless numbers that were supposed to be copied in a particular way. You had to press down hard with the pen."

Her posture and the repetitive motion caused pain in arms and shoulders.

In contrast to the many women who described strenuous labor, Sara felt her job as a teacher was ideal with regard to physical exertion. "I would get up, stand, walk back and forth – no fixed postures, no heavy lifting."

On the farm

A report from the 1930s established that women in agriculture, especially those on small farms, had a heavier work burden than any other group, even compared to men (Nyberg 1989). The most demanding task was the milking, which before milking machines were introduced was done solely by women. They milked the cows by hand and then transported the milk, sometimes a considerable distance. On one occasion Blenda, in charge of the family farm, had been so tired of everything that she had poured out the milk along the way. Only occasionally did she manage to convince her brothers to come and fetch her by horse and carriage or motorcycle. That the milk might go sour was also a worry in the summer. To prevent this it was sometimes lowered into the well, which was strenuous as well as risky.

For women in agriculture, work was also strictly tied to the hours of the day and seasons of the year. The daily routine was set, with milking morning and evening, every day. Summers were especially demanding, with a never-ending tide of both indoor and outdoor tasks. At harvest time, when everyone had to help out in the fields, other work was put aside. "Things a woman was supposed to take care of for herself had to be done before the haying," said Anna. By "for herself" she meant major household tasks that were her responsibility – laundry, cleaning, baking, sewing, weaving, and so on. But she still had to watch the children and her dementia-impaired mother-in-law, do the milking, put food on the table, and wash the dishes. "After the milking I had to help bring in the timothy and clover. It was really heavy going because I was exhausted at the end of the day," she said. Anna also ran a country store that people came to at all hours of the day and night throughout the year. Then whatever else she might be doing, indoors or out, had to be dropped for the moment.

With the advent of milking machines the workload grew somewhat lighter and women were also less tied down, since men not only learned how to operate the machines but also to milk the final drops by hand. For Anna, the constant traipsing back and forth between the house and the fields, the barn and the pasture, home and the store was nevertheless exhausting. "I was always on my feet," she sighed. The hard labor also damaged her health: she was barely 50 when she had a heart attack. The doctor summarized her condition with "You've taken on more than your body can handle." Anna also believed that decades of toil were the cause of her chronic back pain, but in addition she recalled the sense of pride when her strength held out. "When you moved those bags of flour you really flexed your muscles," she commented about work in the store.

Meaning and pride

Despite the negative and strenuous aspects of their salaried work lives, most of the women felt a sense of satisfaction about having contributed something of value to society and their fellow human beings. As the nurse Gertrud related, "My job was fulfilling; that's one of the things that made me feel good and gave me happiness in life." Vera, the engineer, was gratified that she had kept production going. "As I saw it, my mission in life was to keep things running, to make good products we could sell at a profit. During my 35 years at the factory we never dismissed anybody!" On the factory floor, Elna was also pleased about what she had accomplished: "People keep telling me that working in a factory must be the most awful thing you can do. But I enjoyed it. You got a feeling of satisfaction when you had been productive that day. Since the piece rate increased, you also knew it helped everybody." She made an effort to learn how all the machines worked and mastered each step of every operation. Because of this she became a public relations figure at the factory, taking visitors on tours. Not being assigned the same monotonous task all the time also made the days go faster. "When you got there in the morning, you never knew where you'd end up." Another factory worker, Klary, also expressed a sense of pride in one interview when she said, "Let me show you this – I made it myself," holding up a piece of cable braided in a design she herself had fashioned. When her boss later took credit for and profited from her creation, she knew her place in the hierarchy and did not object. Blenda, who ended up working in the municipal home-help service, was content to have had the opportunity to do what she was good at: "Without boasting, I think I'm a caring person. I love taking care of people."

For Sara, the secondary-school teacher, daily challenges were built into her work, which she greatly appreciated: "You had to supplement your knowledge to be ahead of the pupils. That's what I liked – trying to make it interesting and enjoyable for them ... I rarely had problems with the kids." Grade school teacher Marta, in a sparsely populated rural area where the school was poorly equipped – "no books, no globe, no organ" – described how, with the children's help and relying on her own ingenuity, she had been able to acquire everything they needed. This had been a big boost to the children's self-confidence: they had even managed to save enough money for an organ.

Some women were proud of having done a good job at work despite major family responsibilities. Malin, who like Sara had a husband and children and worked full-time, said, "I've been capable, performed well on the job, tried to live up to my responsibilities and make the best of every situation that arises. Tried to see to it that people couldn't come and criticize."

A room of one's own

Salaried work had also given the women a degree of freedom, access to a life separate from their families. Though Malin felt conflicted because she did not live up to the norm of staying home with her children, she also thought it would have been boring to do nothing but take care of the family. "I really appreciated having to leave home in the morning!" she said. Others felt that even the walk or ride to work was a respite, giving them the possibility of "following a line of thought to its conclusion" without being interrupted. For some, the walk also provided fresh air and exercise. A couple of women sometimes worked in another town, which forced a change in domestic responsibilities. As Sara noted, "Then my husband had to take care of everything here at home."

An income of one's own meant increased independence. Irina, previously quite content as a housewife, described this discovery after taking a position as a churchwarden: "When I had a job I didn't need to ask – I had my own money. A fantastic feeling! I had no idea it would feel so good to be a bit independent." For women who were intimidated by their husbands, money of their own provided a degree of power and freedom of action. Greta also noted that in her work as a nurse, the camaraderie among co-workers helped make her private situation bearable. For Elina, who felt isolated and ignored in her marriage, an evening cleaning job offered a breathing space. "I didn't need the money and I never liked cleaning, but it was fun being alone in the evenings, cleaning the offices."

When lack of childcare forced women to stay at home while their children were small, having a job to return to could mean the difference between wellbeing and malaise. Linnea, who suffered from depression during her many years at home, described how much better she felt once she could return to her profession as a physician. "I was so happy to be able to work. It was just fantastic!"

Work and illness

A number of women in the study stated that they rarely missed work because of illness. Estrid, for instance, said, "I was never away from the construction sites – I brought aspirin with me." Neither the women themselves nor their bosses considered fatigue and physical strain acceptable reasons for staying home. Pain or stiffness in muscles and joints were not sufficient cause, either. "Those weren't real illnesses, after all, just little aches and pains you didn't take sick leave for," as Malin said. Before universal health insurance was put in place in 1955,[20] many did not receive economic compensation when ill, a circumstance that was especially difficult for unmarried women. "Every day, every hour you were home, you lost out," said Elna, who was supporting two children on her own. Superiors at work might also have an extremely negative attitude toward absences because of illness; a sick child was not a valid reason for staying home.

Even those who received economic compensation seldom took sick leave. Malin knew it was difficult to find a substitute in the office if she was away. As a teacher, Sara did not think being ill was an option. "Then there was hell to pay later," since she ended up with more to do when she returned. Working on a farm, Anna had a hard time finding anyone to fill in for her. She did the milking as usual despite having pneumonia, and another time went out to the cows immediately after giving birth. Bleeding profusely, she had to manage on her own.

Women working in the healthcare system developed "a tendency to downplay" their own health problems. "Under no circumstances could you let yourself think about that," said Frida, who suffered from a chronic blood disease. Once she had been persuaded to work over Christmas despite being on sick leave. Her comment was, "When you're that exhausted you just keep going – you don't have the energy to deal with it." Linnea also came to work despite being unwell. "I was working insane hours. It went so far that I was on the verge of suicide or psychosis." Without support from her boss she could not

---

20 The new law providing financial compensation during sick leave applied to all salaried workers, and was related to income. A so-called base sum was also paid out to married women without (official) income of their own.

manage to break the vicious circle and kept up the same pace, which led to a heart attack. Greta also described feeling that she could not leave work. "I had a sinus infection, was completely deaf in one ear and had a splitting headache. The doctor sent me home, but I couldn't be away so I came back on the sly."

Several women had managed to work and support themselves despite long periods of illness or other handicaps. They believed, furthermore, that working had helped keep their spirits up and that not letting illness get the upper hand made them stronger. Elna's strenuous and stressful work at the textile factory in all likelihood made her rheumatoid arthritis worse, but after each hospital stay she nevertheless hurried back, wanting to keep her more interesting assignments and be with her co-workers. When she no longer could work, life became dreary until providing daycare for her grandchildren once again gave it meaning. Elina, later in life a preschool teacher, had also stayed in the work force as long as she could despite the hip injury that caused a great deal of pain. "It hurt so much when the kids came running up to me, the way kids do," she said. Still, she loved her work and wanted to continue. It was with a heavy heart that she finally was forced to give it up.

The work environment, not least its social and psychological aspects, was an important factor in helping the women combat illness and pain. Blenda, who since youth had suffered from back pain, pointed out how important it was to enjoy one's job. At one workplace where the atmosphere was unpleasant she had frequently been absent due to illness, while at another where her assignments were similar she had scarcely missed a day – "Probably because we had so much fun together." Britt-Marie recalled that being demoted to monotonous recording tasks led to psychological problems as well as affecting her physical health. "Then I caught a lot of colds and had stomach aches, for the simple reason that I disliked the work." Later, when she once again found a job that drew on her competence, it was "easy as pie" and she was never ill. Marta also found ways to continue working as an artist despite increasingly impaired vision. "When my eyes gave me trouble, I started working with tiny paintings, sat very close and used a magnifying lamp. That's what helped me pull through. I call those pictures my survival pictures," she said.

Retirement

When the women became pensioners the official age of retirement in Sweden was 65, as it remains today. Linnea continued working until this age despite longing for retirement. After her heart attack she returned to work to be accommodating, but for the most part she felt unappreciated and exploited. In addition she was disappointed that her pension was much lower than that of colleagues. "I just hadn't put in all the years you're supposed to." Her husband had never compensated her for the many years she had unwillingly stayed home with children.

Valborg's reaction when a sympathetic doctor enabled her to take early retirement from her cleaning job for health reasons was a sense of liberation. "Not having to wear yourself out was like going to heaven," she said. Klary likewise stopped working at the cable factory before reaching retirement age. After more than thirty years at the same job she was weary and felt it was enough. She also wanted to be at home with her husband, who was retired and in poor health. Other than chronic back pain, she had no serious health problems and never turned to the healthcare system to provide grounds for early retirement. She simply quit, and accepted the economic loss this entailed.

Other women retired earlier than planned for reasons other than illness. Workplaces were reorganized and they were no longer needed. "When no one wanted you any longer, of course you didn't want to stay," said Britt-Marie. When Gertrud left nursing and teaching for a "better" administrative position, she had less influence as well as less job satisfaction. The hierarchical structure of the workplace made her uncomfortable. "You had to take one step at a time, couldn't ever go directly to the person making the decisions." When reorganization opened up the possibility of early retirement, she chose to take it. That was also the outcome for Vera, who toward the end of her career found her opinions ignored and was assigned routine tasks. As her joint problems grew more severe, she decided she might as well retire.

Blenda was among those who stayed in the work force until retirement age. Toward the end of her work life, after many years of toil, she had found an "easy" job providing home care for the elderly. Cleaning and shopping for others was "nothing" compared to her previous work experiences. Edit, who helped run her husband's grocery shop and greatly enjoyed her work, continued past retirement age. When the shop was sold she took a part-time position in another store and did not stop working until age 72.

An adequate pension

A number of the women had to get by on very small pensions, in particular those in poorly paid lines of work and those who had stayed home with children for long periods.[21] For some whose husbands were still alive, economic dependence was even greater after retirement. For others with long periods of dependence on their husbands' money, the pension, perhaps the first fixed income in their lives, could mean a new feeling of self-determination. This was the case, for example, for the farm wife Anna and the housewife Karin. As a widow even Edit, despite a low income from work in her husband's grocery, was rather well off; she had "inherited" a portion of his pension, a provision that remained in place for women in this generation, based on the assumption of a single provider per family.

Valborg, on the other hand, with a low pension from cleaning work, found herself in financial straits because her husband, after years of homecare, had been moved to a care facility. Most of his pension was charged for the fee and little was left for her to live on. She always worried about daily expenses, especially unexpected ones. Her social life, even contact with her children, and activities outside the home became severely limited. Best off after retirement were those who, like Vera, Sara, and Malin, held relatively well-paying positions in the regular work force for many years.

---

21 A universal pension law was enacted in Sweden in 1913. Since then the pension system has been revised several times. In 1935 the scale became the same for women and men, but only after 1948 was the base pension large enough to live on. For the women in this study, pensions were based on the number of years in the work force, annual income during the final five years, and sometimes a supplemental occupational pension according to union contract. Pensions now are based on lifetime earnings, with supplemental occupational and private insurance. There is still a base pension for those who have minimal earnings or none at all.

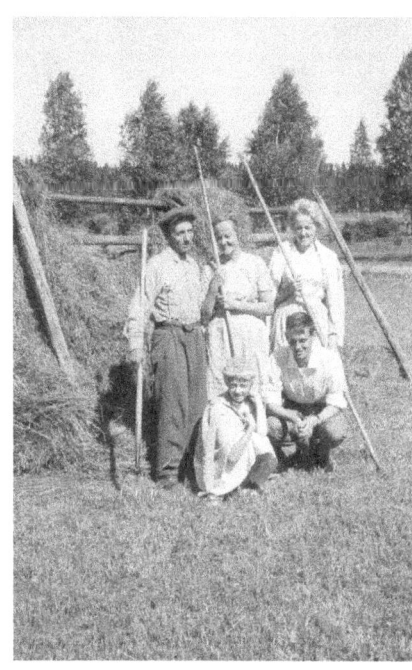

Annika Forssén (crouching) with her parents and two of her siblings at the hay-drying rack – 1960s.

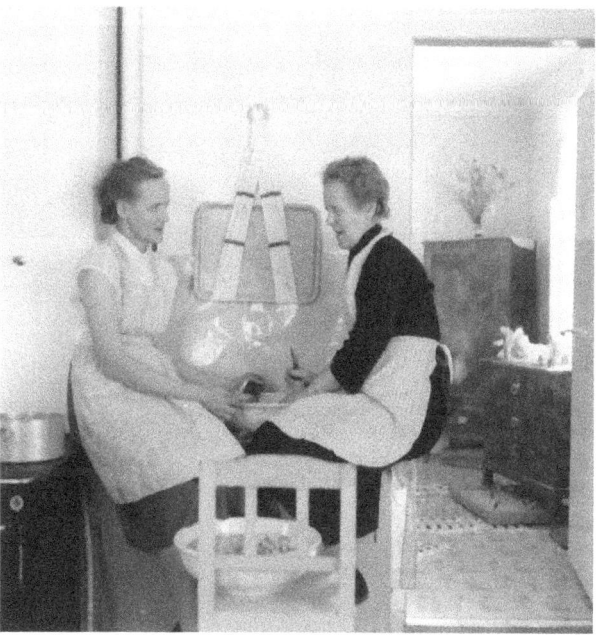

Annika Forssén's mother and her sister-in-law preparing the Sunday meal – 1950s.

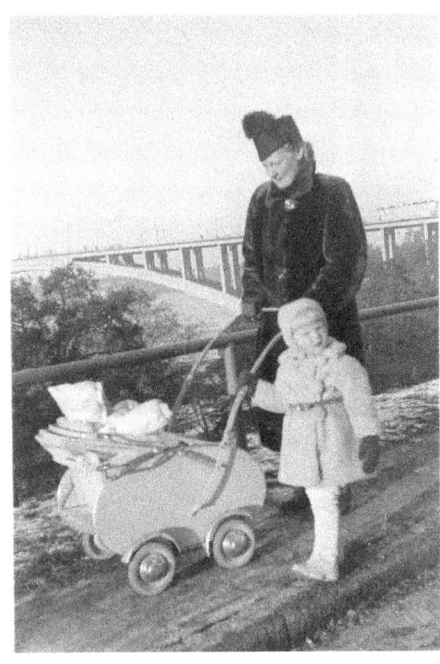

Gunilla Carlstedt's mother with two of her children out for a walk in their home town – 1940s.

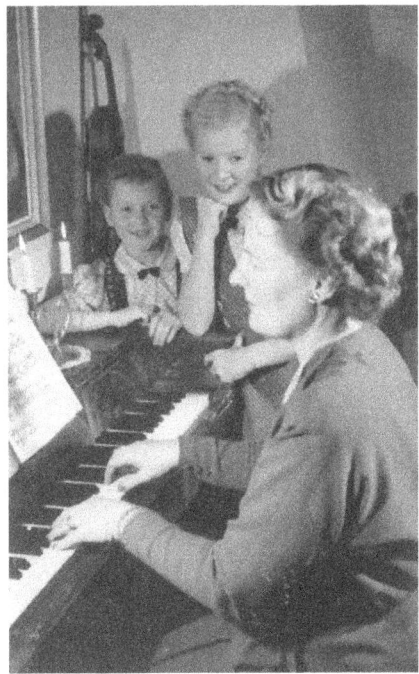

Gunilla Carlstedt (right) and her sister listening to their mother playing the piano – 1950s.

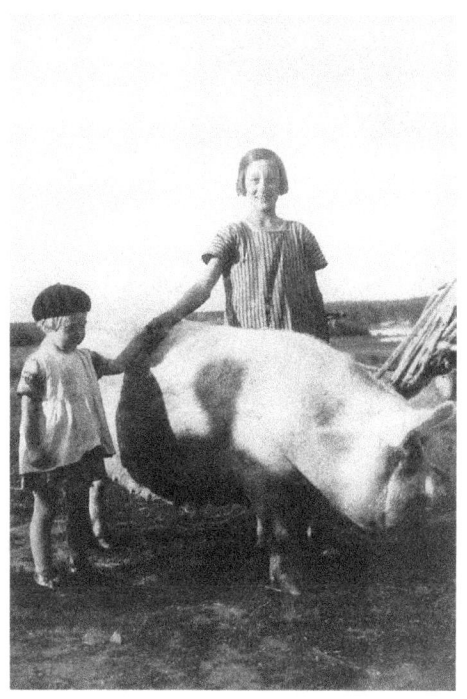

Anna as a twelve-year-old foster child.

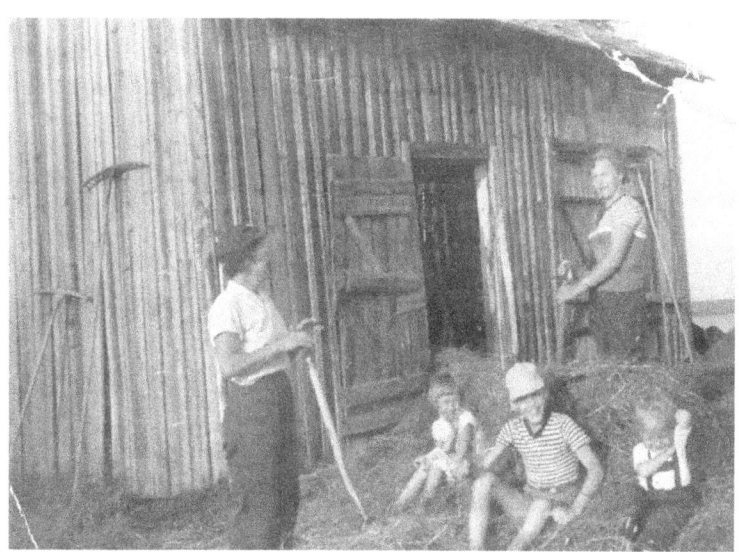

Anna cutting hay – 1950s.

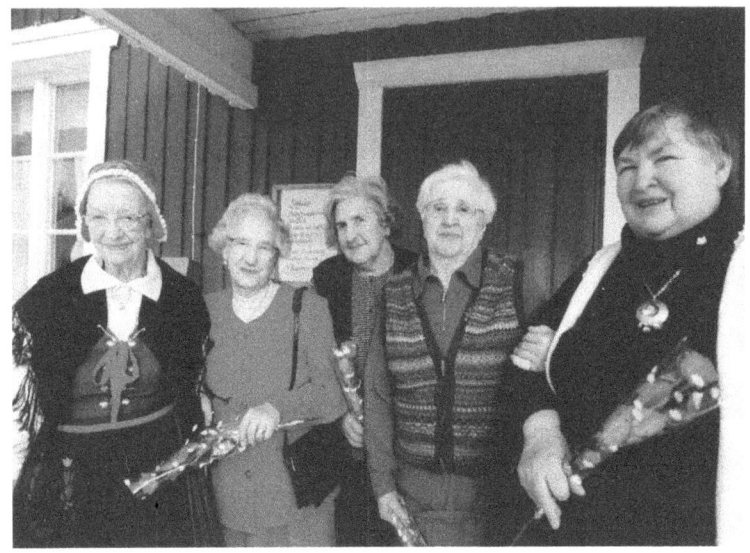

Anna (second from left) with members of the Housewives' Association – 1980s.

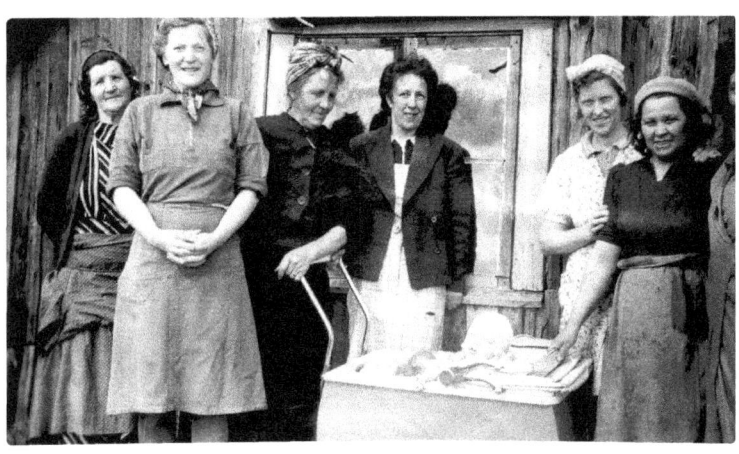

Blenda (in the middle) on the island where she grew up with her daughter and women neighbors – 1945.

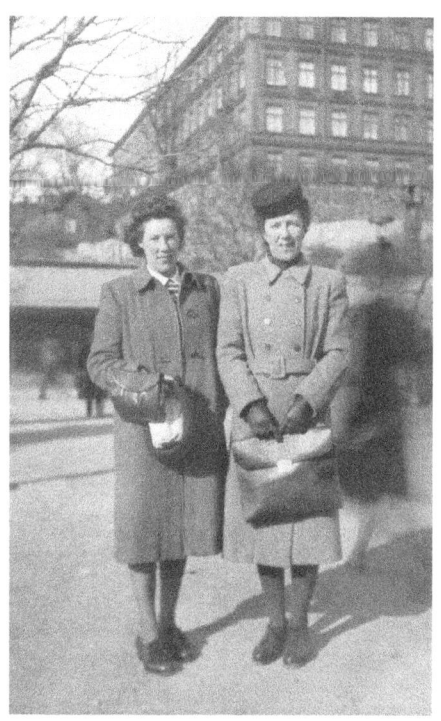

Blenda (right) and her sister on their way to the municipal library – 1940s.

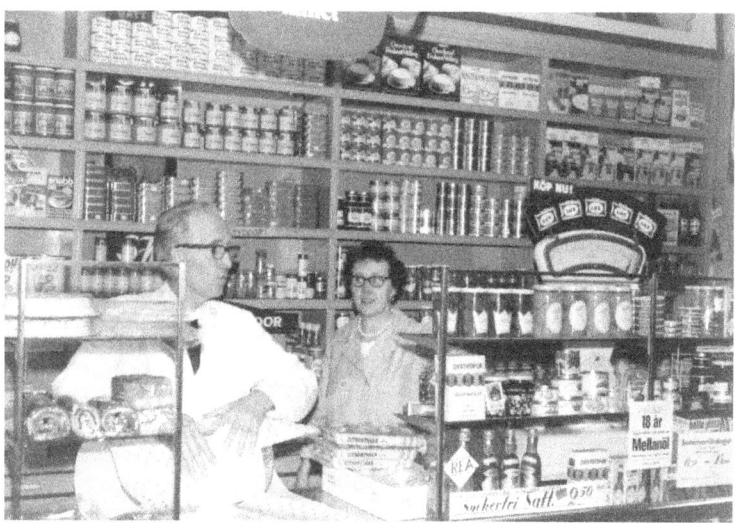

Edit and her husband in their shop – 1970s.

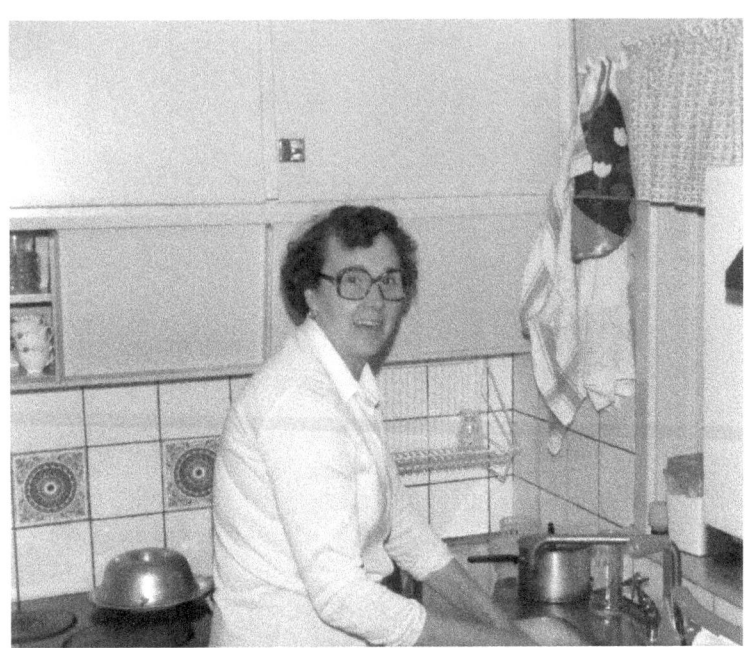

Edit at home in her kitchen – 1970s.

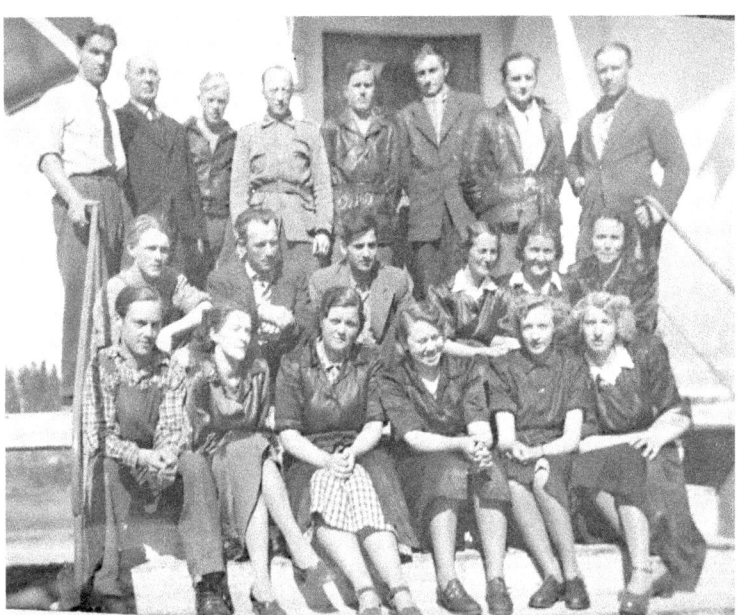

Elna (bottom row, second from left) with co-workers at the textile factory – 1950s.

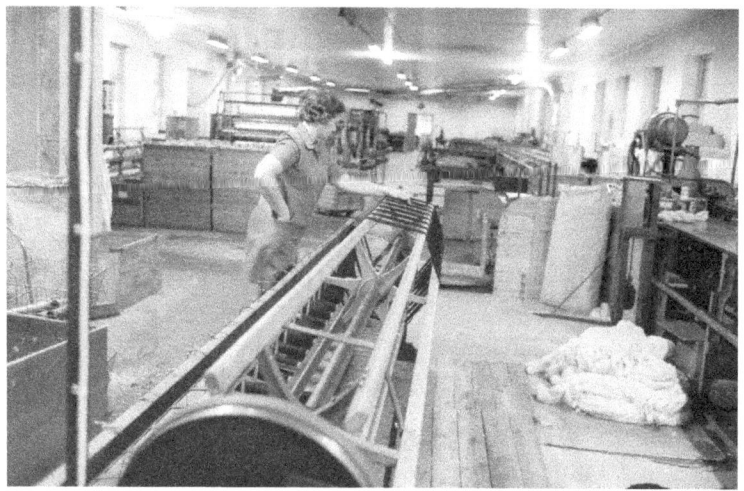

Elna's work station at the reel in the textile factory – 1970s.

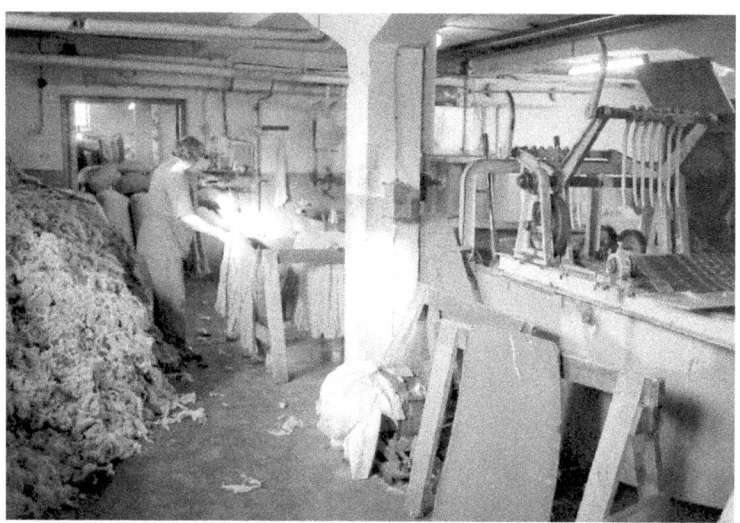

In the cellar of the textile factory – 1970s.

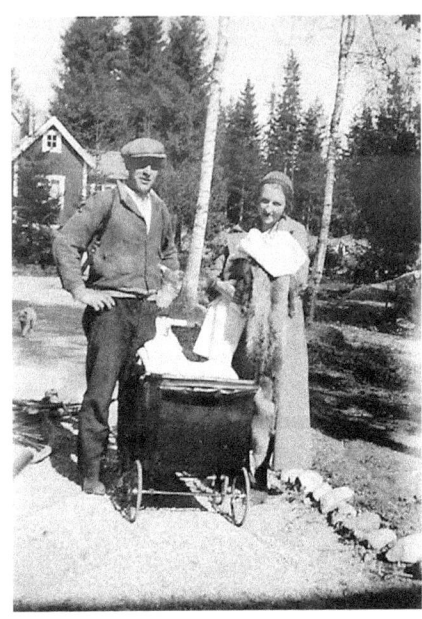

Estrid with husband and children outside the home they built themselves – 1930s.

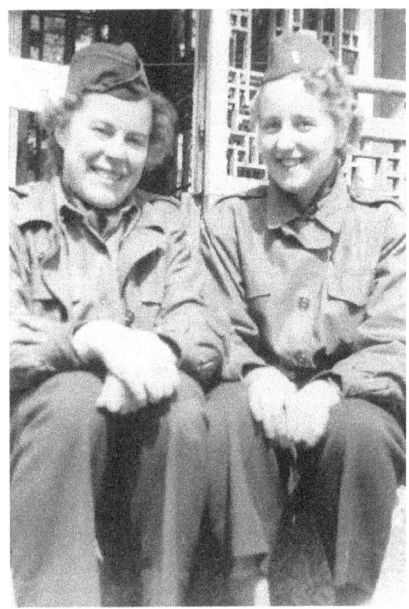

Gertrud (right) as an aid worker during the Korean War – 1950s.

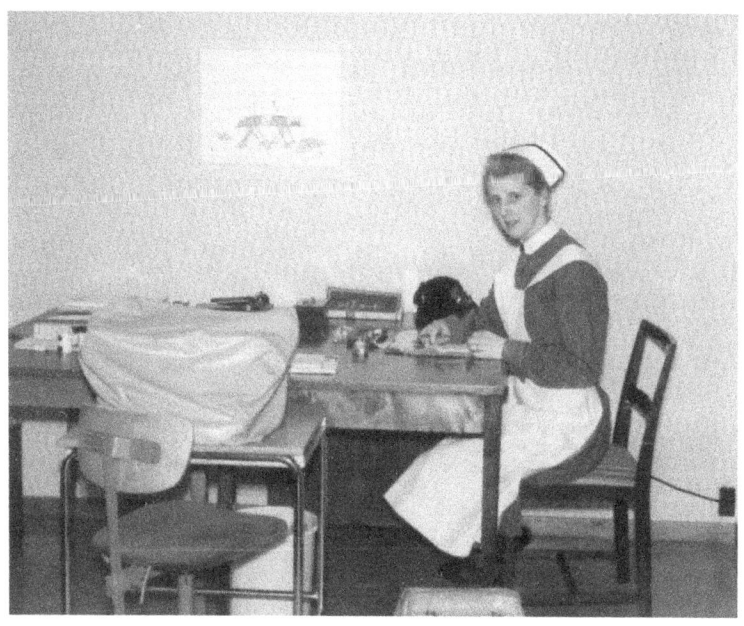

Nurse Gertrud at her workplace – 1960s.

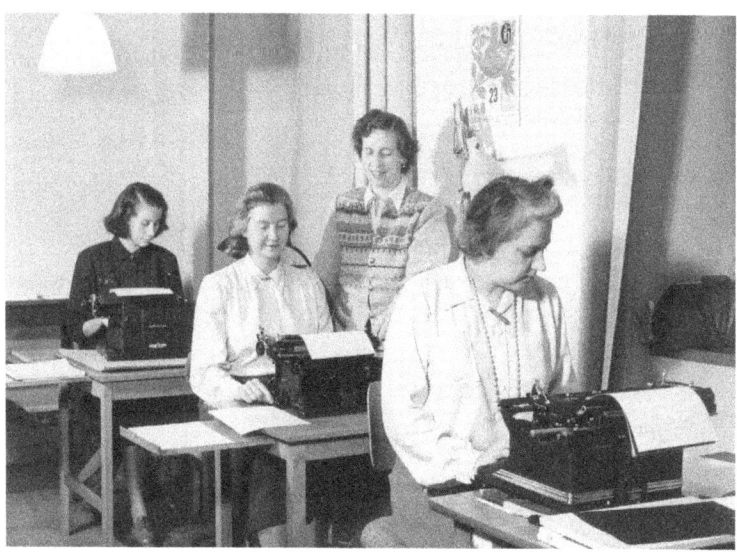

Malin (standing) in charge of office staff – 1949.

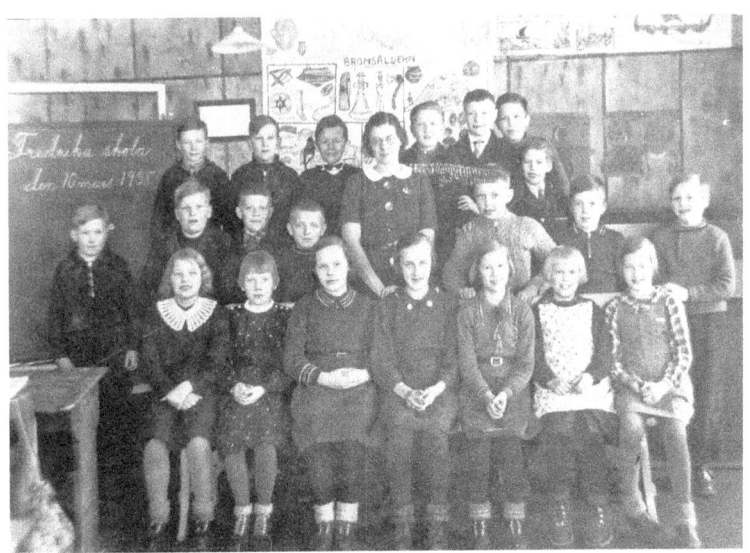

Marta with her pupils – 1938.

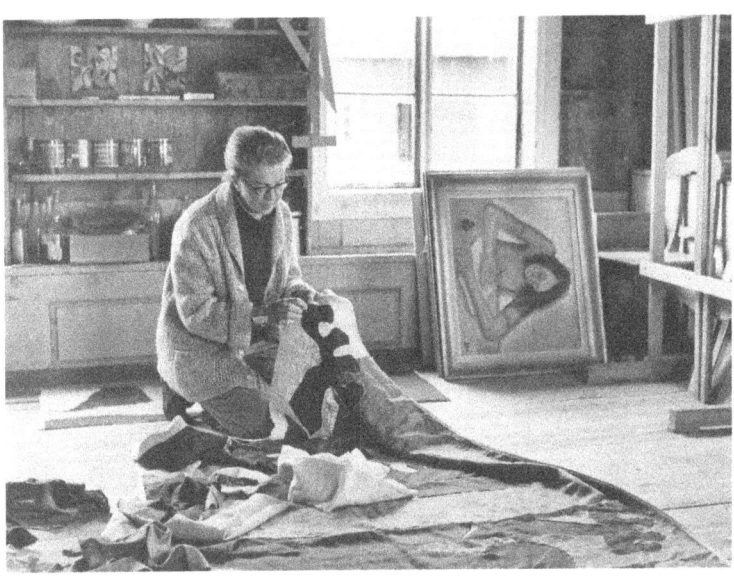

Marta in her studio – 1960s.

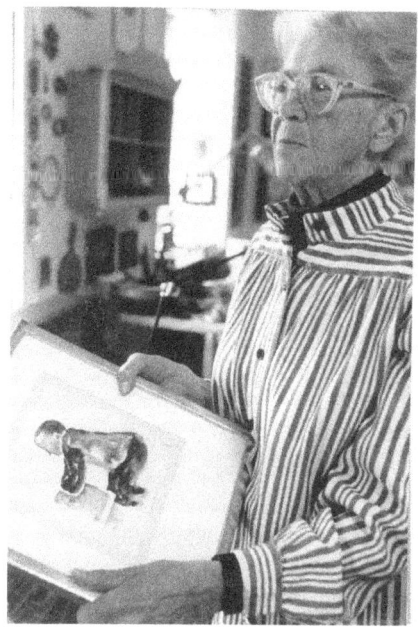

Marta late in life with one of her watercolors of children – 1990s.

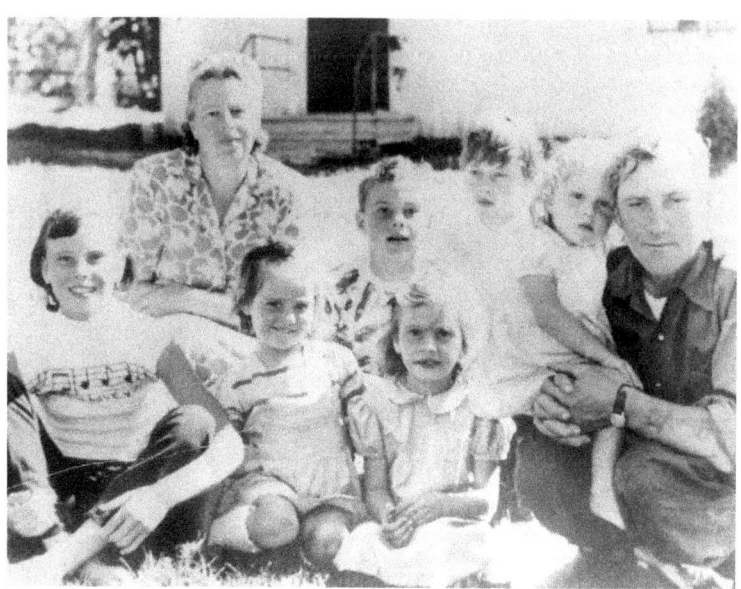

Signe with her husband and some of their children – early 1950s.

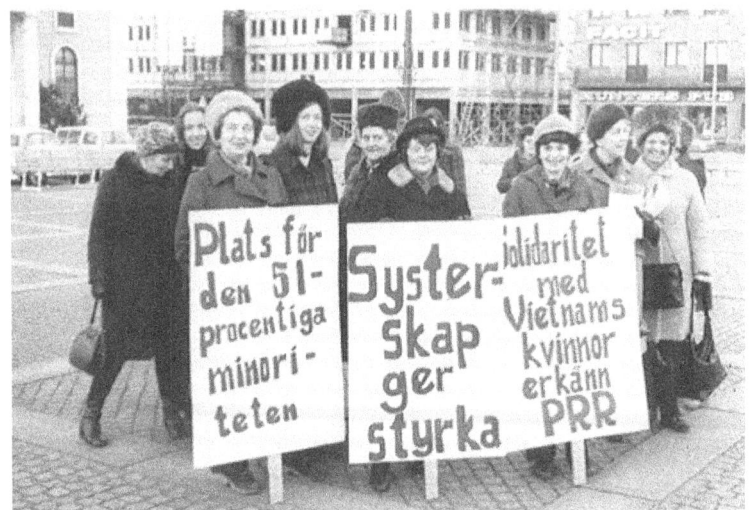

Women's political organization in which Signe was active. The signs read (left to right): "Make room for the 51 percent minority"; "Strength in sisterhood" and "Solidarity with the women of Vietnam. Recognize PRR." – early 1970s.

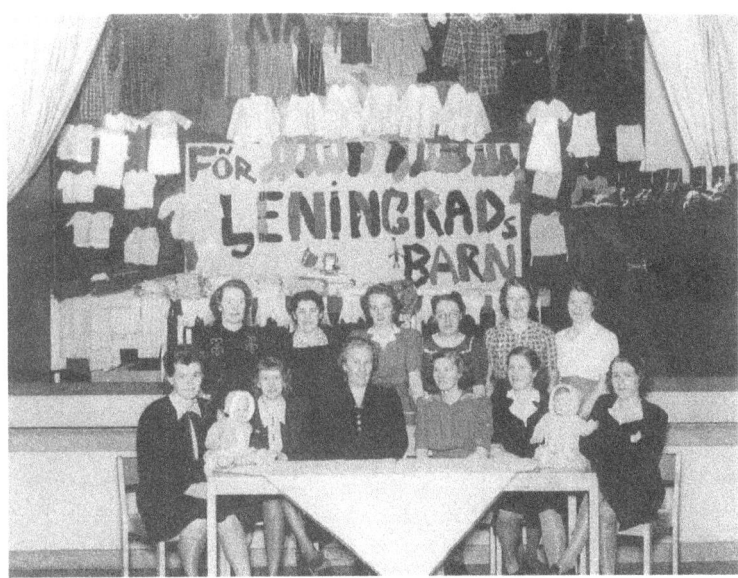

Women's organization providing assistance to child victims of war – 1940s.

7

Health and Illness

The welfare state and public health

During the 1910s and 1920s, when the women in this study were born, the greatest threat to health was infectious disease. Several participants had witnessed, for instance, the decline and death of siblings or parents from tuberculosis. Beginning in the 1930s, however, major changes occurred. The political effort to create a welfare state included, in addition to better housing, improved diet and nutrition for large segments of the population and an increase in the level of education. Universal cost-free healthcare was implemented in 1955. In just a few decades, these reforms, along with advances in medical science, dramatically improved the likelihood of surviving illness and maintaining health. In the 1940s, when effective medicine to treat tuberculosis was introduced along with a vaccination program, this disease was drastically curtailed. The introduction of penicillin, also in the 1940s, enabled treatment of common illnesses such as pneumonia, childbed fever, and scarlet fever. A vaccination program against diphtheria, polio, and tetanus virtually wiped them out. Once insulin could be artificially produced, diabetes was no longer life-threatening. The median life expectancy in Sweden increased rapidly, from about 60 years in the 1910s to more than 70 at mid-century.[22]

During the second half of the twentieth century, so-called diseases of prosperity such as cardiovascular disease and cancer replaced infectious disease as the leading causes of death in Sweden, as in the rest of the western world. Cardiovascular disease struck men and women in more or less equal measure, but women were (and are) more likely to be affected later in life. For middle-aged women, the leading cause of death was cancer, in particular breast cancer. Between the ages of 15

---

22 Subsequently it has continued to rise, to nearly 82 in 2012 – 84 for women and 80 for men.

and 44, the most common causes of death for both men and women were cancer, accidents, and acts of violence, though young men were (and are) three times more likely than young women to die in accidents or through violence.[23]

Class-based differences in health and survival rates at the turn of the twentieth century diminished after the mid-century mark but subsequently began increasing again.[24] Difficult life circumstances have always been associated with a higher risk of cardiovascular disease. Deaths from this cause were fewer in the last decade of the century, but the shift was most apparent among men.

Throughout the century, movement disorders such as rheumatoid arthritis and other conditions causing pain and diminished mobility have affected large groups of women from middle age on. Many women, young as well as old, have also suffered from psychological disorders in the form of anxiety and depression (Socialstyrelsen 1991, 2001; Statistics Sweden 2012). Migraine and urinary tract infections have also limited the daily lives of many women, as have handicaps such as poor vision (Socialstyrelsen 1991, 2001).

Strong – but fatigued

The women's perception of their health was closely correlated to how they had managed the tasks and responsibilities that fell to them. When they mentioned "being healthy," the words "having the strength to work" often followed. Malin, who was responsible for supporting her family, commented on her health over the years as follows: "Don't think I gave much thought to my energy level or whether I was well. Being strong was the only option." Even if the women were ill, furthermore, the demands on them often remained the same. As they saw it, the line between being sick and being well was whether or not they were confined to bed. "You were never sick, stayed on your feet no matter what. The only time I was flat on my back I had pneumonia," said Karin.

---

23 This is a major reason for the shorter life expectancy of men, since risk-taking, for instance behind the wheel of a car, is part of the norm for "masculine" behavior in much of the world (Phillips 2005). Work-related accidents are also more common among men.

24 In 2012, highly educated individuals lived an average of 5 years longer than those with little education, though the class differential was greater among men than women. The calculation is nevertheless complicated by the fact that women's actual class identification is more determined by that of their spouses than is the reverse.

Though they felt strong and accomplished a great deal, the women were fatigued, often for extended periods of time. They spoke of this as a normal condition, saying they'd "gotten used to it" and that "all women were tired." "Of course I was tired all the time, exhausted," said Sara, referring to the years when she was employed full-time and had small children at home. Signe remembered, "I was extremely worn out, exhausted at night and when I got up in the morning." With expressions like "you take a deep breath" and "you pull yourself together" the women described how they nevertheless had done what was necessary.

For married women, the husband's attitude affected the workload – some women received support and assistance when they were exhausted or ill, whereas others received little or no help. Regardless, everyone emphasized that they never complained, to their husbands or anyone else. "I never admitted I was tired and down," said Anna, who like many others pushed herself to the limit to meet expectations. She had not even protested when her husband took a job away from home, leaving the entire responsibility of running the farm to her. Only once had she complained that the demands were unreasonable. "You know how much I have to do, you know I don't have the strength to work after 8 p.m.," she had told her husband.

Sara felt let down because her husband did not share household responsibilities but had given up, expecting neither change nor concern for her wellbeing. "I've had a very hard time of it, but I'm healthy and strong. Haven't ever complained, you can't do that. You have to accept the way things are." Linnea, who had been taught as a child that she should "be there for others," described "denying and ignoring" warning signals from her body. She thought this capacity for denial was reinforced in her marriage, where she felt more and more isolated. "It's meaningless to focus on yourself. No one listens, so there's no point in exploring how you feel – nothing changes anyway." Not taking illness, pain, or exhaustion into account might also be seen as a matter of principle. "Am I really that lazy?" Valborg thought to herself in the laundry room when she felt done in. She then fainted and was found to have double pneumonia.

Women whose marriages were unhappy described a particular type of fatigue. "You had to watch out," said Elina, always on her guard against her husband's unpredictable temper and behavior. Rest and a good night's sleep did not cure this kind of weariness. Greta described her exhaustion as "vanishing into thin air" when she had the opportunity to get together with others outside the home.

Exhausted due to illness

Frida suffered from a serious blood disorder and recurring ovarian cysts that necessitated abdominal surgery and radiation treatment. She was extremely fatigued, but was nevertheless expected to manage working at her nursing job as well as caring for her husband and mother, both of whom were in poor health. When her condition was most acute she received excellent medical care, but subsequent periods of sick leave were brief. Eventually she realized that the only alternative was to quit her job, a decision reached in desperation: "I had nothing, had no idea what I'd do, but I simply didn't have the strength." The loss of income caused difficulties for the family and she herself became financially dependent on her husband. Much later, when Frida received a disability pension, the diagnosis – despite her illnesses and caregiving responsibilities – was "psychological deficiencies."

Some women were so accustomed to fatigue that they did not realize they were seriously ill and needed medical attention. Anna mentioned that farm work had left her "tired to the bone" for several years before she had a heart attack around age 50. On the evening it (presumably) occurred, she was on her way home from a meeting in the village. "I ended up sitting in a snowdrift, just didn't have the strength to go on. Later I crawled home, ate something and slept. The next day I went about things as usual. I thought I was just exhausted and overworked."

The physician Linnea also misinterpreted signs of fatigue and thought her chest pains came from the neck. Consequently it was a week before she went to the hospital, where it was determined that the symptoms had been caused by a heart attack. She was still exhausted when she was released. Despite strict orders about what she was and was not allowed to do, no one asked whether there was anyone at home to help her – and there was not. When she mentioned at a checkup that she suspected she suffered from heart failure, no one listened.

Elina spent a week in bed, paralyzed by fatigue, but even after that things did not improve. "I had chest pains while I was weaving, had to sleep halfway sitting up, snored and had a dry cough." But at the healthcare facility no one took her account seriously or wanted to examine her. Instead the doctor advised her to build up her strength through exercise. "I tried to bike, but it wore me out." It turned out that she had had a heart attack and now was suffering from angina as well as heart failure.

At about age 60, when Greta sought treatment for fatigue, the physician interpreted her symptoms as post-menopausal. Hormone treatment caused problematic bleeding before it was determined that the cause was a defective heart valve.

"Aches" – and pain

Many women suffered from pain, often chronic. This was often referred to as an "ache," and like fatigue was regarded as a normal condition, in part because it could not be allowed to get in the way of what needed to be done, in part because the healthcare system had not assigned a diagnosis to the symptoms. "All women experience some pain – most of the ones I know do," observed Sara.

Headaches were common; for relief, the usual recourse was pills. Edit, who suffered from migraines, could nevertheless rest during work hours thanks to her position as the boss's wife. "I said, now you'll have to get along without me for a while. I can't read the scale." Pain in muscles and joints was also common. Elina, the preschool teacher with an injured hip, was in chronic pain and wanted to have surgery. "An operation isn't called for, and there's no need for X-rays," said the doctor. When X-rays eventually were taken, they revealed serious damage to the hip joint, but rather than being remitted for surgery Elina was placed on sick leave. The years that followed were dominated by pain and despair. "What sense is there in making people suffer this way?" she burst out. "When I was cleaning at home I couldn't stand up – I sat on the floor while I wiped it. Sometimes I was so exhausted that all I could do was sit on the edge of the bathtub and cry." Throughout the ordeal she missed her work, which she had greatly enjoyed. Only when the social insurance agency wanted her to undergo job retraining did she finally, four years later, have surgery, but by then it was too late to return to her former job.

Estrid likewise was forced to wait a long time for treatment. Both knee joints were worn out, causing pain and difficulty in walking. "The doctor thought I could get by with canes," she said. For years she used two sticks to navigate – to the store and back, on the bus, and in public places. She was past 80 when, after repeated appeals, she finally had surgery.

When Elna first developed rheumatoid arthritis around age 45, she thought the symptoms were caused by muscle strain, but the doctor saw it as a work-related injury typical for her type of work operating a spinning machine. He nevertheless did not prescribe a change at the workplace or arrange for sick leave, but rather provided her with elastic bandages. Greta, the district nurse, suffered from wrist pain caused by years of recording information by hand. This was not, however, classified as a work-related injury, but as a post-menopausal condition – the same misdiagnosis she later received when she had a defective heart valve.

By the time of the interviews, Signe's body ached and she had chest pains, but after many years of trying to get help she had given up. "It isn't worth the trouble to mention my pains to the doctor. He doesn't listen anyway, just gets irritated," she said. This anticipated lack of response meant that she never expressed what she was thinking and wanted to say. For her and others like her, the physician's perceived unwillingness to listen meant that prescribed treatment could be experienced as inappropriate and that medicine was not always picked up at the pharmacy.

Gynaecological "problems"

Symptoms or problems relating to the reproductive organs or to hormone-related physical changes made the line between health and illness, normal and abnormal, especially difficult to draw. The women described their menstrual periods in strikingly different ways, from "not especially bothersome" to "extremely painful." Several had suffered from heavy bleeding. On a couple of occasions Signe had such a low blood count that she fainted, but she was also the one who felt stronger whenever she was pregnant. For many years after the birth of her last child she had "terrible" bleeding, but she did not want to have a hysterectomy, since she had heard that made you "old and nervous." Her fears derived from the then-prevalent medical practice of removing "everything," including the ovaries, which quickly brought on menopause.

For a number of years Sara also suffered from heavy menstrual bleeding. She was 38, a full-time teacher, wife, and mother and was convinced the bleeding was stress-related. Despite her relatively young age a full hysterectomy was recommended to remove the ovaries as well as the uterus. Looking back, she remembered her shock when the doctor joked that soon she'd be rid of all her internal sex organs. "Won't it be nice to be done with all that, he said." Sara experienced the comment as "appalling."

Most of the women did not mention ordinary menopause as having been especially problematic. Some "didn't remember," a few had hot flashes, another recalled perspiring a lot. Karin remembered that she "could get irritated," but beyond that had not had any problems. In fact, it worried her that she did *not* have any. Was she truly normal? Irina, who had neither heavy bleeding nor any other difficulties, was nevertheless told she should have a hysterectomy. In her upper middle-class circle women often underwent this procedure when they reached menopause. After the operation she felt dreadful but was never given an explanation: the sudden, drastic reduction in hormone levels. She received no hormone replacement therapy, only tranquilizers that made her ill. On her own initiative she stopped taking them, but it was a long time before her body adjusted.

Britt-Marie, the youngest of the women, had taken hormones during menopause. After a few years she stopped, wanting to see if she really needed the pills, and decided she did not. No one in the healthcare system, however, had suggested that she go off them.

Several women recalled occasions when they had felt vulnerable and embarrassed in connection with gynecological examinations. Without being asked, Elna was confronted by an entire group of male medical students who were to be present during the examination. When the professor stepped out of the room for a moment she was left on the examining table, her feet in the stirrups. The students started making joking remarks about her private parts, using Latin words they assumed she would not understand. She did understand, however, and remembered the incident as deeply offensive and humiliating.

A number of the women suffered from prolonged, recurring urinary tract infections or incontinence but felt their condition had seldom been taken seriously by medical professionals. "I've been in such terrible pain," said Valborg, "but they couldn't find a cure, only temporary relief." Klary also suffered from chronic urinary tract infections, which made it difficult to work since she had to make frequent trips to the toilet located in another part of the factory building. Even so, she was never given sick leave. Urinary tract problems, in particular incontinence, could also make women worry about the future, as Gertrud declared with the words "I don't want to be an old lady who wets her pants."

Mental illness

Several of the women had suffered from psychological problems. Britt-Marie had been hospitalized and on medication for anxiety and depression, symptoms that were brought on by relationship breakups and bullying and lack of respect on the job. As time passed she learned to manage her symptoms and was able to go off medication. Though she was ashamed of being ill, she also conveyed a sense of self-respect: "I've never dumped my problems onto anyone else. I haven't been dependent on anyone, and I've been able to support myself."

Linnea suffered from depression and chronic fatigue, which she felt was caused by her heavy workload as a psychiatrist and by her sensitivity to her patients' situation, something she had deliberately cultivated. Without support from colleagues and superiors, she struggled for years "to survive." In the end it was anger that saved her. "No one is going to put me down," she had started thinking. Greta, who had "really let myself go" due to many years of psychological abuse, found the strength to assert herself through psychotherapy. "I had to find out what it was about myself that made things turn out this way. I have to protect myself – that's what I'm working on," she said.

A number of the women had periodic sleep disturbances and were prescribed tranquilizers or sleeping pills. After using them in moderation for many years, Irina started feeling weak and anxious, which made her question her pill intake. Instead she tried, as did others, to have a bite to eat or to make the hours pass by reading, listening to tapes, or solving crossword puzzles.

Medical treatment

Disappointment dominated the women's accounts of the medical establishment, but they also described receiving good care and being treated with respect and consideration. When diagnosed with bladder cancer, Blenda had felt great anguish – "I walked around the apartment screaming," she recalled – but her fear of dying had let up once she was hospitalized and receiving care. Others shared this feeling of being in good hands, regardless of the illness. They remembered the medical staff as caring and having an eye to their particular needs. "They were really good to me, the girls at the hospital," said Valborg, for example.

Some found it especially gratifying to encounter a woman physician. "It was a relief when female medical students asked you all those questions," said Elna. "She was wonderful – it was like talking to my mother," was Estrid's description of one physician. The chronically exhausted Frida recalled being treated by a female psychiatrist as her most positive experience in the healthcare system. She had encountered respect for her struggle to function in daily life and felt the doctor understood her situation. "It was fantastic to meet someone who thought it was amazing I'd been able to manage at all!"

Several of the women were helped by physicians who realized that their illnesses and symptoms were caused by overexertion at work or, conversely, made it difficult to perform on the job. This happened, for instance, to Valborg, the cleaner, who was put on sick leave for an entire summer with the diagnosis "weak heart." Work had left her exhausted and she needed the rest, but she did not believe she suffered from a heart condition: "The doctor saw how worn out I was."

When Anna, the farm wife, had a heart attack the physician took it as a given that her workload was too heavy. "I wasn't supposed to do a thing. 'Your husband will have to help out,' he said." When the social insurance agency initially granted only a 50 percent disability pension, claiming she was still able to manage some household tasks, the physician once again backed her up. Anna did eventually receive a full disability pension. Contributing factors may have been that the work of farm wives began to be registered as full-time employment at this time and that the farm had to be sold when Anna became ill

Elna's contact with doctors left her with mixed feelings. She recalled with gratitude one occasion from the time when she had small children and was working several jobs. "The doctor saw that I was undernourished and exhausted and put me on sick leave for several weeks." At that time a period of rest gave her a much-needed respite. Later in life she felt differently when another doctor, without asking what she preferred, arranged for a disability pension. "I guess he had good intentions," she said, "but that wasn't what I wanted – I wanted job retraining." Though she protested, her rheumatoid arthritis meant that she was considered completely incapable of working.

Caring for others

The women also came into contact with the healthcare system when caring for ailing family members. A number of them had found it difficult to make their voices heard, despite the fact that they had taken on primary caregiving responsibilities – Frida, Gertrud, and Valborg when their husbands were in poor health and Linnea raising her handicapped son. They also felt that their own situation got no response from the healthcare system. "It would have been nice if someone had just wondered how I was doing," Frida remembered thinking as she shuttled her husband between hospital and home. She was the one who had "tennis elbow" (an inflamed tendon) from pounding on his back to loosen phlegm from his diseased lungs. Even those who themselves were old when working as caregivers felt ignored by the healthcare system, despite the fact that their freedom was restricted and they often were exhausted or suffered injuries from heavy lifting.

A dominant precept of medical science at the time, that bad mothering was the cause of both physical and mental illness in children, caused distress for some of the women and led to feelings of guilt. Linnea felt called into question as a mother and realized that she alone would be responsible for planning her son's future. Signe was criticized for not allowing her children to be inoculated with untested vaccines. The commonly accepted childrearing regime – breastfeeding every four hours, no bottle feeding, not picking up a crying child – also made life more difficult for some of the women, as their stories made clear.

Maintaining health

The women had made a deliberate effort to maintain their physical and psychological wellbeing. Over time they had learned what was needed. For some, a sense of humor and "taking pleasure in the little things" in social interaction and at work were essential. "To feel good, I need to be playful and teasing and be around others who are," said Elina. A number of women also pointed out the necessity of having time for themselves. Sara, for instance, would sometimes get away and become incommunicado by taking the train to town and going to a café. "Nobody knew where I was and it felt like such a luxury to be alone!" This kind of escape was not possible for everyone, but the women were well aware of their needs and most of them could find strategies to be alone for a while. Anna pointed out the importance of Sunday church services and the expectation that "Sundays would be a day of rest."

Many women also felt the need for beauty and sensory pleasure and made music, art, and literature a significant part of their everyday lives. For Frida, dancing was absolutely vital; it had helped her summon the energy to face her many operations. "Dancing to jazz music was pure bliss – that really brought me to life. When I hear the right kind of music I want to dance all by myself." Two women played musical instruments, others sang in choirs or listened to music. "German Lieder – that combination of text and music, without it being opera. It's so magnificent, oh, just fantastic!" exclaimed Britt-Marie. Books were very important to most of them, especially reading for a while in the evening despite being tired. Some chose entertaining books for relaxation, others preferred material they could identify with.

Being outdoors in nature was a source of joy and serenity; working in the garden revived body and soul. Even indoors there were small, everyday pleasures. "Won't you admire my flowers?" asked Klary after an interview. "I think they're lovely, and the birds outside my window keep me company."

The women were aware that nutritious food and regular exercise were essential to maintaining health. "I've taken care of myself, exercised, eaten healthy food at regular times," said Karin, who had always taken part in exercise and dance classes. "I've always walked from home to school rather than taking the bus – an active, healthy lifestyle," said Sara. Not everyone, however, could take exercise classes or "eat right." Those who were single parents and/or poorly paid were periodically short of food and had neither time nor energy for particular exercise activities. Physical exertion on the job or walking or biking to work was all they could manage. Valborg nevertheless recalled a small window of opportunity she had managed to find. "I used to go out on my bike on Sunday mornings – it was great," she said. In sum, options for taking care of oneself physically were dependent on social class, financial circumstances, and the way the marriage functioned.

For some women, discussion of "maintaining one's health" awakened guilt feelings and shame, in particular for those who were battling weight problems. Regardless of the cause, excess weight was seen as self-induced, by the women themselves and by those around them. "I know I'm too fat and eat too much of the wrong things. Maybe I needed to hear that my blood sugar was too high," said Greta. The physician Linnea held herself responsible for her heart attack. "I've been a chain smoker, and that was a contributing factor. I have only myself to blame."

In old age

At the time of the interviews some of the women were still dealing with exhaustion, pain, and illness. Despite being past 80, Valborg continued to care for her ailing husband at home. "My head starts to spin and I feel dizzy. The last time I jumped up at night when he called I fell against the sofa. Hit my chin and my knee. Does my life really have to be like this?" she burst out in distress.

Several of the women suffered from eye diseases or vision problems that led to limitations in daily life, such as not being able to read, watch television, or do handiwork. Worst off was Marta, the artist, who had gone almost completely blind. Concerning work, her great passion, she said, "Of course it's an impossible situation for a painter to lose her sight!" She tried to keep her spirits up and fill her days meaningfully by listening to books on tape, taking walks in her familiar neighborhood, and getting together with friends. "Well, I'm alive, and I'm not in pain. But if I needed help all the time and just sat twiddling my thumbs – that would be hard. Then I really wouldn't want to go on."

Edit, who was partially paralyzed after a stroke, could no longer go out alone. "I miss that! But you have to get used to it, not being able to do a lot of things." Even so, she did exercises regularly and hoped she would improve. "I can feel I'm getting better, starting to regain my strength. Once the weather improves, we'll go outside!" Regular visits from homecare services gave a number of the women a sense of security, but financial cutbacks loomed. For a time Edit's alarm was taken away. It was returned to her only after she had fallen several times without being able to call for help.

Estrid was also afraid that if she needed help it would not arrive in time. She had joint problems, poor vision, and diabetes and periodically had to make emergency trips to the hospital due to atrial fibrillation (a heart disorder). She gave the following contradictory description of her condition: "Things are fine as long as I stay reasonably healthy, though actually I'm sick, of course. But I won't die for a while yet – I'm peppy and feel good physically." For her, loneliness was the worst complaint, and getting out to see others was the only way she could combat it. Emphasizing her healthy side thus became a survival strategy. Many things were also the matter with Blenda, but she did the same: "I'm almost, almost always healthy. My aches are the kind of thing I pay no attention to. My life right now is very full."

Signe pointed out one precondition for wellbeing that applied to many women: "It's important that your children stay healthy, and you yourself to some degree, if you're going to feel all right."

8

Looking Back, and Ahead

Contentment and sorrow

When the women looked back, a number of them felt that overall, in spite of everything, their lives had been good. "I had a hard time of it, but I took pleasure in my work," said Anna, though she also mourned the endless toil: "When I walk across the meadow now I think, Goodness, how hard I worked here. It makes me sad." It was Anna who had heard from the doctor that "You've taken on more than your body can handle." Greta likewise testified that her daily work encompassed both pleasure and drudgery. "I can certainly say I've had a full life, but sometimes it was just too much." She was also sorry that her work at the rectory never was recognized and that she had stayed for so long with a husband who browbeat her. We also recall Valborg, who grieved over a life without love and kept longing for a few words of appreciation from the husband she took care of. Toward the end of her life she was worn down from exertion and disappointment.

Several of the women whose husbands were still alive described sharing good experiences. "I have my husband, who asks for me," said Irina. "Every day at 3 p.m. we drink coffee made the Hungarian way – it's our little ritual." In contrast, others worried that the possibility of "a life of their own" would diminish over the years or that they would not have the strength to provide care if their husbands were ailing. Some wondered what would happen if they themselves became ill. Would their husbands be able to give them the care they needed and hoped for? A number of women also worried about illnesses that would affect their intellect or personality or were concerned that they might become dependent on and cause difficulties for their children.

The women who were widows and missed their husbands and their lives together nevertheless felt they were doing well. Thus Edit felt secure about having been loved and could take pleasure in her memories as well as her current life. Others who had felt appreciated for taking care of ailing husbands could enjoy a newfound freedom; they had done everything in their power to assist their mates and could now live as they themselves chose. After her divorce, Linnea likewise felt good about being on her own. Now that she was alone, she could restrain herself from "always putting others first." Signe also enjoyed the solitude once all her children had moved out. "Just think, being able to sit by myself and drink coffee," she said, describing quiet mornings with lighted candles.

Two women who had always been unattached or had not cohabited with their partners saw being alone in old age as positive. As mentioned previously, the artist Marta worked best during solitary evenings. In retirement Vera thought it was lovely to "read the newspaper in peace and quiet" in the morning without the stress of hurrying off to the factory. Britt-Marie, living alone and with no close relatives, had a different reaction. The prospect of growing old in isolation, of being forced to get help from strangers, of dying alone, filled her with "an indescribable dread."

Women who had experienced a great sorrow found that it never let up. Two who had lost their mothers when they were young felt this had impacted their entire lives. For those who had endured the death of a child, the pain never went away. The two women who had lived through war, Elina from Finland and Irina from Hungary, also found it difficult to look back. "I certainly didn't want to live the life I've had. The war – it ruined my entire life," said Elina, though 50 years had passed since that time. Irina also had intense memories from the war years and from the post-war Soviet occupation. "We lived in terror every day – we stood at the windows, watching the bombs fall." Everything the family owned was destroyed and later her husband was arrested. "It was during Stalin's rule. I'll never forget the fear whenever the doorbell rang. My God, who could it be? The secret police?"

Self-recrimination and shame

Faced with difficulties and failures, the women often assumed the blame. They regretted attitudes, actions, and choices, and might admonish themselves even for matters they could not control. Others had also placed a burden of guilt on them or done nothing to discourage this response. "This has always been my worst enemy – that I can feel what others feel," said Valborg, and continued, "You bring misfortune on yourself!" – referring also, and once again, to the baby that had died at birth. Toward the end of the interview period she was no longer responsible for the daily care of her alcoholic and sickly husband, but was still unhappy and felt things were amiss. She was weighed down by guilt feelings about her husband's placement in a care facility against his will and visited him daily, though this exhausted her because all he did was complain. "The children are angry with me. They want me to have a good time now, relax and enjoy life, and not visit him all the time. But I can't break the habit of identifying with him and feeling his pain!"

A number of women felt they had allowed themselves to be intimidated and cowed. They blamed themselves for keeping silent, for avoiding conflict or not setting clearer boundaries for what others could expect of them. This was Sara's experience. After the birth of her second child she had dropped out of graduate school, having lost the necessary drive and self-confidence when her husband questioned her competence. Afterwards she felt "awful" about it. Linnea always lived with the feeling that she "wasn't good enough," despite signs of professional success: "I somehow never measured up in my own eyes – that little piece was missing inside me." One way of handling this feeling was to live up to her own and others' expectations as a wife and mother and refrain from getting divorced or working in the profession she enjoyed. In retrospect she felt she had been "a coward," had "let herself be exploited" and had channelled her anger in a self-destructive manner by smoking. "If I hadn't smoked I'd have rebelled much earlier," she said.

Britt-Marie sometimes mentioned that she felt she was "a total failure" because she had neither managed to advance professionally nor to maintain a relationship with a man. Vera and Blenda had periods when they saw themselves as ugly, in both cases because their mothers had communicated this to them. Only late in life did Vera understand the reason: her mother was ashamed of her own Sami background and appearance, which was held in contempt where she lived. For Blenda, the issue was that she had never felt her mother liked her.

Reconciliation and hope

As they aged, however, a number of the women began acting more autonomously, without paying as much attention to what others thought. They accomplished things they had never thought possible: arranged to live alone, found new jobs, developed new interests, and protested against injustice and lack of respect. Linnea, who had gotten a divorce and broken with friends she felt had taken advantage of her, had discovered a stance that helped her move on: "I need to rely on my intuition – then things go fine," she said, though she also regretted not having put her foot down at work before chronic fatigue and heart problems set in. Greta said, "I still feel insignificant, but I've elbowed my way up – I'm no longer so unsure of myself in polite society." Vera had written a letter to Swedish television protesting the derisive portrayal of single women. "Why should we old maids be presented as nastier than other people?" she asked.

Several women mentioned the need to write – poems, letters, diaries, short memoirs and occasionally articles on topical issues. They wrote to make themselves seen and heard, by others and by themselves. Writing also led to reflection. "You have to express what's inside you – they can read about it when I'm gone," said Estrid. For some, music became a way to express their feelings. Greta related, "I visited a good friend who was sick and played something on her piano. She enjoyed it even though I made mistakes. I think that was the turning point, that someone wanted to listen to me."

Meaningful, positive changes in life also included improved finances and housing. By now all the women had modern conveniences at home; those who had toiled without them were glad they no longer had to bring in water and wood or shovel snow. Blenda related that every day she thought, "God, how wonderful it is to have this cozy little place." She was also among those whose financial situation had improved in old age and could now afford things that were not absolutely essential: "I open the closet and look at my clothes. Just think, to be able to buy something that's pretty! In the past everything I bought was on sale."

For some, reconciliation with fate and with the way life had turned out alleviated bitterness and sorrow. "All wounds will heal," Malin had taught herself to think over the years. "When life is difficult, I still think things will pass," said Vera. Feelings of guilt and failure could be counterbalanced by pleasure and pride about significant ways in which they had "been useful," whether in private life or on the job. Thus Gertrud, despite having been caught between responsibility for the household and her work as a nurse, now felt good because she was "satisfied about what she had accomplished." Similarly, Estrid had dealt with money problems as well as her husband's periodic drinking bouts but felt gratified that she nevertheless had been able to give her children a good home.

Several of the women found particular solace in their Christian faith, which provided "meaning and a goal" and "the perspective of eternity," as Vera expressed it. Blenda felt that she was one of "God's grandchildren" and church had been "a home" to her. "When I return to the church of my childhood I'm flooded with memories – funerals, baptisms, confirmations and all. Religion was the core of our upbringing

– Dad was a churchwarden and Mother was deeply religious as well. You can't wash that away – it's a part of you, deep, deep inside."

At the time of the interviews the women still communicated longing and hope and thought about what they hoped the future would bring. Several looked forward to more extensive contact with relatives and friends. Others were caught up in everything they still wanted to do, see, and learn. They dreamed about traveling, taking courses, improving their language skills, pursuing cultural activities, reading or making music. As Greta put it, "I'm not going to die yet. I still have so many things left to do."

Part II: Analysis and Discussion

Introduction

In Part I of the book, study participants spoke in their own voices. In Part II, we place their narratives in a more theoretical context and relate them to women's situation in Sweden today. We begin with childbearing, separated from other forms of unpaid work due to its unique character and the exceptional significance the women assigned to it. In the following chapters, focus is on unpaid work of other kinds, paid work, and medical attitudes to women's illnesses. Finally, we return to some of the common symptoms and strategies for health revealed in the women's stories.

9

Childbearing as Work

Initially we did not view childbearing as particularly central to our research project. During the interviews, however, the women spoke at length and with great intensity about, first and foremost, their experience of labor and delivery, their contacts with prenatal clinics and the care they received on maternity wards. At first we did not listen very carefully, especially when they discussed labor and delivery. We thought an event that lasted a few hours or days was of minimal interest in our investigation. We aimed to highlight other types of work the women had performed and wanted to counter the focus on reproductive biology that often characterizes research on women's health. Our perception was also colored by our profession as physicians, for whom childbirth without medical complications is considered "normal" and therefore "uninteresting." Most likely we were also influenced by prejudices conveyed in medical school: the belief that women often exaggerate when they describe their experience of giving birth. Only gradually and after the women returned to the topic time after time did we understand that childbirth – how well they thought they had managed it and how they had been treated – had major significance for their wellbeing throughout life. This also made us reflect on our own experiences of childbearing and the work it entailed.

Passive language and active work

Once we had processed the idea that pregnancy, giving birth, and breastfeeding are work, we became aware of the perceptions conveyed by language use – and what it hides. To emphasize that pregnancy and childbirth require physical and emotional energy we would like to replace passive expressions like "to be expecting" and "having a baby" with more active terms such as "bearing and nourishing" and "giving birth" to a baby. Referring to "the work of childbearing" can also make it easier to view the conditions women encounter – for instance with regard to prenatal care and care during labor and delivery – as work environment issues.

If we add up the time the women in our study spent at childbearing work, including breastfeeding, we find that the woman who bore ten children devoted approximately twelve years to this physical labor. For a number of the others it was five or six years. The woman who had many miscarriages, then gave birth to a baby that died at birth and finally to a baby that survived had four years of childbearing work behind her to produce a single child. This type of work was largely invisible to others. Being pregnant is furthermore associated with physical symptoms such as nausea, back pain, and exhaustion. It can also be risky, for instance in cases of pre-eclampsia or hemorrhage, and strenuous in the last trimester. The women in our study described long-lasting illnesses associated with pregnancy, including urinary incontinence, hemorrhoids, and back and pelvic pain.

Viewing childbearing as work also draws attention to conditions for pregnant women in other work situations. Many of the women we interviewed had worked hard at both unpaid labor and salaried jobs during their pregnancies. They received no special consideration because of their condition, and some of them connected fatigue, miscarriage, and infant mortality to this fact. Their circumstances resembled those that many impoverished women across the world continue to encounter. Heavy lifting at work causes increased risks during pregnancy. In present-day Sweden women in certain physically demanding occupations have the right to paid leave in late pregnancy, compensated at the same rate as sick leave. The definition of heavy work, however, is still under discussion. The caregiving professions, with heavy lifting and/or physically and psychologically stressful night duty, are ordinarily excluded.

Assignment of sick leave during pregnancy has shifted several times since the mid-twentieth century; sometimes it has been more readily available, at other times less so. The situation of an individual woman has depended on social standards, but also on varying practices in different geographic locations and the personal sentiments of particular doctors.

Prenatal care and women's responsibility

As previously mentioned, during the early decades of the twentieth century pregnant women were assigned a large share of the blame for the high infant and maternal mortality rates of the period, despite the fact that women had been denied information about their own bodies, sexuality, and the process of giving birth. The establishment of cost-free prenatal clinics, beginning in the 1930s, brought great improvements in medical care for pregnant women. Along with other political efforts to promote economic security and good health within the framework of the welfare state, this led to a significant decrease in infant and maternal mortality rates in subsequent decades, with Sweden's becoming among the lowest in the world.

The medical profession's increased control over childbearing was simultaneously accompanied by an authoritarian attitude toward women who were pregnant or in labor. In particular, those women who previously had managed these matters themselves but were now expected to follow the dictates of the experts, could encounter problems. Their own knowledge and experience was ignored and many felt they were belittled and disparaged. For one woman in the study who was called into question this way and did not return to the prenatal clinic in her next pregnancy, the decision was fraught with peril. She hemorrhaged in the delivery room, which soon became life threatening because she was suffering from untreated anemia. But even women who followed doctors' orders were not always treated with respect, which made them less likely to seek medical care and consequently led to increased risks for both mother and child.

From the mid-twentieth century on, most women in Sweden have followed the recommendation to receive care at a prenatal clinic. In recent years, furthermore, many have come more often than is medically necessary. The usual explanation given is that women of today are less sure of themselves. In our opinion this perception needs to be seen in relation to the fact that they encounter more information and must take more factors into consideration than was previously the case. They are screened for more risk factors and markers, leading to worry and sometimes necessitating difficult decisions. Their lifestyle with regard to nutrition and exercise is examined and they hear about the risks associated with increased levels of chemicals in the environment and in food.[1] Most women make a great effort to follow the recommendations they are given. However, expectant fathers are less involved in discussions of nutrition, despite the fact that men – as the women in our study noted – have a major influence on the family's diet. It is likewise only expectant mothers who are tested for sexually transmitted

---

1 In Sweden, pregnant women and more generally women of childbearing age are, for example, discouraged from eating fatty fish from the Baltic due to the high level of dioxin, while at the same time fatty fish is promoted as a very healthy food choice.

diseases; the healthcare system ignores the possibility of father-to-mother-to-child infection during pregnancy. Primary responsibility for the health of the unborn baby is thus assigned to the individual woman. The father's responsibility is glossed over, and it is up to the woman to deal with the effect of stress at work or environmental risk factors.

The attention directed toward pregnant women and their unborn babies in Sweden and other prosperous countries is in stark contrast to the lack of interest impoverished women encounter in poor countries and in countries where economic resources are less evenly divided. About 20,000 women die every day from pregnancy-related complications associated with poverty. The Egyptian professor of gynecology Mahmoud Fathalla asserts that "Women are not dying of diseases we can't treat. They are dying because societies have yet to make the decision that their lives are worth saving."[2]

The lifelong effects of dismissive treatment

Some women in the study recalled the experience of childbirth with pride and elation. They felt they had received the help and care they needed, at home or in the hospital, and that giving birth was unproblematic. Their memories were intense but positive. For the majority, however, the memories that dominated were painful. These women felt they had not lived up to others' expectations, or their own, of how they would perform. In conversations with us their memories of fear, desperation, and powerlessness resurfaced. Several described incidents during labor and delivery that we consider physical and psychological abuse. This was the first time these women had told anyone about what had happened half a century earlier. Their long silence testifies to the feelings of shame and failure associated with these memories.

Previous research has established that the experience of giving birth has a long-term effect on a woman's psychological wellbeing. Twenty years on, a positive experience increased a woman's sense of self-worth while a negative experience had the opposite effect, and moreover the intensity of the effect increased over time (Simkin 1991; 1992). The prolonged symptoms resembling those of post-traumatic stress described by one woman in our study were triggered by disrespectful treatment and a sense of complete defenselessness after she had given birth. Her story was reminiscent of those told by

---

2 http://www.amnestyusa.org/our-work/campaigns/demand-dignity/maternal-health-is-a-human-right.

victims of sexual abuse. Her reactions after the incident were also similar: a sense of shock; the inability to tell anyone about what she had undergone; fear that no one would understand, since the baby was healthy; guilt feelings; a sense of not being like others; and an effort to make everything go on as usual, as if nothing had happened. For this woman, breastfeeding became agonizing because it aroused feelings of apprehension and panic connected to her post-delivery trauma. That she nevertheless continued nursing the baby was most likely an attempt to meet the expectations for being a "good mother" to compensate for her previous "failure." This undisclosed suffering and a sense of being inferior to other women had followed her throughout life and she never became pregnant again. That the experience of childbirth, even today and in medically uncomplicated deliveries, can be conveyed in "a language of rape" and lead to consequences similar to those described here has been confirmed in other research (Kitzinger 1992; Beck 2006, 2011; Thompson and Downe 2008).

One woman, blamed by healthcare staff for the death of her baby at birth, was plagued by self-recrimination and guilt feelings for the rest of her life. In a previous stay on the maternity ward she had been admonished about making a fuss, so she did not dare request a Caesarean section, which might have saved the baby. Other women remembered being called into question during labor and delivery, abandoned at critical junctures and subjected to painful procedures. As we see it, stitching a vaginal tear or incision without administering anesthesia – which was common practice – should be considered abuse. The women were shocked and taken aback when this occurred but had also learned to be accommodating to avoid further maltreatment.

Participants in our study were not chosen on the basis of their experiences during childbirth, yet many of them stressed difficulties associated with it. Research on younger women suggests that although trauma is uncommon, experiences similar to those of the women we interviewed are shared by younger age groups as well. Our work as physicians also supports these findings; we have encountered women who suffered in silence for decades from anxiety and guilt associated with the birth of a child.[3]

---

[3] For additional information and references, see Forssén 2012.

Norms and expectations

Most of the childbirth experiences the women in the study remembered with such distress had been medically normal, that is, without medical complications. Labor and delivery had also been in accordance with the prevailing understanding of what "natural labor" entailed, which meant no anesthetics were administered. Natural labor – vaginal delivery without anesthesia – is also recommended today, but an effort is made to listen to the preferences of the women themselves, to take their anxiety and fear seriously, and to provide support during and after labor, making childbirth a positive experience for many women. Traumatic experiences nevertheless continue to occur at a rate of about 7 percent in Sweden (Waldenström et al. 2004), caused in large part by a sense of disempowerment and a perception that the staff is indifferent and uninvolved (see Forssén 2012). Present-day cutbacks to the healthcare system may make negative experiences more common as women encounter stress when hospital space is inadequate and the staff is under enormous pressure.

Many women are afraid of "failing," or think they have failed if technical intervention becomes necessary during labor and delivery (Beck and Watson 2008; Beck 2011). They may also feel pressure to remain calm and focused and be anxious about "losing control." These and other factors contribute to a general fear of giving birth that in recent decades has become more widespread among women in Sweden and the western world. It is a common perception that this fear is a main reason that the number of Caesarean sections has increased, which is viewed as a negative development both from a health perspective and in terms of cost. The increased number of Caesareans in Sweden and elsewhere has multiple causes, however, several of which weigh much more heavily than the woman's preferences or "convenience." Factors include physicians' attitudes; advances in technology that can lead to surgical delivery "just in case"; type of facility (there is a higher rate of C-sections in private rather than public hospitals); types of economic compensation in the healthcare system; insurance questions; and norms within the family and social network (Bewley and Cockburn 2002; Villar et al. 2006; Högberg 2013).

Breastfeeding today is also affected by norms similar to those described by the women in the study. A number of them had pressed on despite painful sores on their breasts and despite an inadequate milk supply. One woman who had stopped breastfeeding early felt guilty about not giving her baby the right nutrition and saw a connection between this deficit and her daughter's eating problems as a teenager.

In our practices we have also encountered women who express this kind of self-recrimination and anxiety when they have not managed to breastfeed as prescribed. We believe it is important to lighten the burden of guilt in these situations. Breastfeeding has a very limited significance for a baby's health in prosperous countries like Sweden, where clean water and breast milk substitute (formula) are readily available. Instead social and economic factors are most important for a baby's future good health.

10

Unpaid Work

Living in a family constellation with husband and children led, as we have seen, to women being allotted, or voluntarily assuming, total responsibility for meeting the everyday needs of other family members. This was in accordance with the gender norm of the period and applied whether or not a woman had salaried employment, even if she was the primary breadwinner. For single mothers, responsibilities encompassed every aspect of life and were very labor-intensive, not least due to financial constraints and lack of childcare. Work in the home included a broad range of duties, everything from providing a listening ear and promoting family harmony to cleaning the house, washing piles of laundry, preparing elegant dinners and welcoming guests. Sometimes the women also, willingly or not, took on tasks that traditionally fell to men, often strenuous ones such as shoveling snow, while it was rare for men to help with household chores or childcare. Women who did not have salaried jobs came to see work in the home as their primary mission in life. A couple of those with outside employment also considered it natural, "pretty much inborn," that they were the focal point of the home, the organizer and manager. Others had fought a long battle with their husbands for a shared workload and responsibilities. Two of them eventually grew tired of the imbalance and inequality; one got a divorce and the other moved to her own apartment. Two others had avoided this kind of inequality by not marrying.

Mothers become home-nurturers

The Swedish philosopher Ulla Holm examines the reason primary responsibility for the household has come to fall so exclusively to women, not just women in this study, but most women (Holm 1993). Her starting point is childbearing. Being pregnant, giving birth, and breastfeeding, all tied to the female body, she calls "mothering".

Caring for the child in other ways not connected to the body she calls "nurturing".[4] The difference between the two is that nurturing can be done by someone other than the biological mother.

Most women who give birth to children will also nurture them. The concept encompasses caregiving, fostering relationships, and running the household; consequently there is a slippery slope from mothering, which is biologically determined, to nurturing or "home-nurturing", which requires social and practical skills. Frequently this has also been regarded as biologically determined, a view that remains common today. Although present-day Sweden is considered one of the world's most egalitarian countries with regard to gender issues and many men now are involved in caregiving and housework, there are still far more women than men who are responsible for seeing to it that home-nurturing work gets done. Expectations for women, their upbringing and the role model provided by their mothers have often made them more familiar with these skills than men are when their life as a couple begins. This leads to women taking on or being assigned the role of work coordinator within the home, with the result that tasks not expressly allotted to someone else end up in the women's purview (Magnusson 1997; 2005; 2008). Another issue is that others often hold women responsible for the way the household is run and the children are brought up, regardless of who actually does the work.

Unseen work

Much of the work the women in this study did in the home was not visible to outsiders and was not considered real work. This particularly concerned the planning and organizing necessary to make everyday life run smoothly for all family members, encompassing finances, shopping, meals, time schedules, the children's schooling and leisure activities, and so on. Caregiving also involved matters that went unnoticed, such as alertness to dangers, attention to needs, and listening. Many of these tasks were dealt with simultaneously. Women have often been thought to have a natural talent for multi-tasking. The stories these women told demonstrate that they were forced to acquire this competence because everyday life demanded it.

Establishing and maintaining social relations is another unseen task, not least supporting the external social networks of individual family members and the family as a whole. Previous research of long

---

4 In the original Swedish, Holm uses the verbs "mödra" and "modra", both invented terms derived from the noun "moder" (mother).

standing has shown that frequent, meaningful contacts with a wider circle have a positive effect on the health of everyone in the family (Lewis et al. 1976). Many women had been trained from childhood to work on relationships – a skill closely connected to caregiving – by watching older women interact with others and through their own work with siblings. In their adult lives, one important aspect of this type of work was holding the family together and keeping spirits up. There was strong social pressure to assume this role; newspapers and the radio informed women that this was their "duty as citizens" and that it was their own fault if they failed (Hirdman 1987). Many women in the study considered themselves responsible for creating a pleasant atmosphere in the home. To achieve this, and to have some peace and quiet, they had often kept their own preferences and opinions to themselves. Mediating between fathers and children was another task the women had taken on to avert arguments and maintain domestic harmony.

Caring for family members in the home and providing emotional and practical support to other relatives and friends might promote the health of the recipients but was rarely seen as work. Daily care was often necessary, for instance of elderly parents, and might encompass visits, phone calls, and letters. In interviews, the women described how this work could completely wear them out, though in time management studies it generally falls under the category of "leisure activities."

Housework: specialized and strenuous

It often goes unnoticed that many household tasks require technical skills. The term "technological work" is frequently applied restrictively to activities that traditionally have occupied men, such as work in a machine shop, as an automobile repairman, or as an electrician. There are, however, many technical aspects to working with household equipment, using a sewing machine or setting up a loom, all of which require knowledge of how the equipment operates and to what end (Waldén 2001). This work, especially if it is unpaid, nevertheless has neither the same status nor is considered to require the same (professional) skills as technical or mechanical work primarily performed by men.

When all work within the home was considered "women's work," even the most arduous tasks fell to women. The presence of a man in the household could make the workload heavier, since women brought in water, firewood, and food for him. Given that men, on the average, have 50 percent greater strength in their arms and upper body, many of the most strenuous of the women's chores would have been more suitable for their husbands.

Over time, the overall improvement in standard of living – above all in housing, with the availability of running water, central heating, and washing machines – made the work less physically challenging. Geographic location, social class and the husband's attitude nevertheless determined the rate at which the women gained access to modern amenities. Those with the fewest economic resources had, and continue to have in Sweden today, the poorest and least practical housing; their time was also, by necessity, devoted to finding inexpensive merchandise and mending and patching things for reuse. Since standards of personal hygiene and the expectation that clean clothes will be available have steadily increased, the time that women spend doing laundry for the family has not diminished as much as is often assumed (Nyberg 1989).

Family size also impacted the burden of labor. The assumption has always been that women who bear children will be able to care for them without help from others, regardless of how many children there are. The mother of ten in our study, widowed when the youngest child was only a few years old, received neither financial nor practical assistance from outside sources and was left to get by on her own. Today there are still no guidelines about how much unpaid childcare it is reasonable to expect someone to handle alone. Most families in Sweden have two or at most three children and society is organized around that pattern. This may make it difficult for women with many children to find models for how to manage caregiving and work in the home as well as salaried work outside it.

The husband as a work task

The accounts of married women bore witness to the way running a household easily grew to include personally waiting on their husbands. The "marriage contract" many had entered into, endorsed by their husbands and society at large, was that the wife was expected to prioritize the marital relationship and caring for her husband, while he was expected to put primary focus on his salaried work. For some women, caring for their husbands was self-evident and intrinsic to their love for them (compare Jonasdottir 1991; Magnusson 2005). In a number of cases, however, the one-sided nature of services provided led to husbands becoming so dependent on their wives that they no longer could manage their daily lives on their own, whether it came to practical and emotional matters or their health.

As early as the 1930s and '40s, the sociologist and public voice Alva Myrdal described how women's work as housewives and childcare providers had expanded to include adult men, as this passage in one of her articles illustrates:

> Even in modern companionate marriages when both husband and wife often work eight hours a day in salaried positions, it is still considered "natural" that the woman in addition takes on not only all the work in the shared household but also the care of her husband and his possessions. This demonstrates how easy it still is to conflate womanliness with the most taxing aspects of housework. (Myrdal 1938: 29)

Little had changed thirty years later, when a female member of the Swedish parliament characterized the husband in an "ordinary" Swedish family as follows:

> ... somewhat brusque and very preoccupied by his work and perhaps his hobbies. He is inclined to make most family decisions, is lost in the kitchen and a bit bewildered about how to stay neat and clean, a little awkward when it comes to expressing feelings, but deep down he has a good heart. He feels tenderness for his wife and is her biggest child. (Eriksson 1964: 19)

In the 1980s, another expert on women's issues called the personal services that married women provide their husbands "care of healthy husband in the home" (Bolin 1987).[5] Throughout the twentieth century and beyond, feminists and politically active women have thus drawn attention to and problematized the way men (mis)use women as housekeepers and personal attendants. Yet the pattern of the woman who serves and the man who demands service has endured. It is especially pronounced in relationships where the man is domineering, physically violent or emotionally abusive.

The demands on women were even greater when it came to caring for ailing husbands. Despite being aware of the already existing imbalance, it was difficult for them to refuse to take on such caregiving responsibilities: that would make them look like "bad wives." This caregiving was often characterized by heavy physical labor, additional housework, time constraints, and less time to oneself. The quality of the relationship and whether the woman felt acknowledged and

---

5 Bolin's formulation alludes ironically to the legal provision that working parents receive financial compensation for "care of ill child in the home."

appreciated for her efforts had a great impact on how this duty was experienced.

Many older women in Sweden continue to assume an equally heavy work burden, and the situation is not likely to improve. Since the majority of married or cohabiting women have older partners, the task of caring for a spouse around-the-clock in the home is more likely to fall to women than to men (Danielsson and Lindberg 2001). In addition, women in Sweden and worldwide are caregivers at a higher age than men and for longer periods; those they care for are sicker and their own health is worse (Yee and Schultz 2000; Danielsson and Lindberg 2001). Men who care for family members usually receive more assistance from outside sources and at an earlier stage than women in comparable situations. Older women who live alone – a large group, since many married women become widows toward the end of their lives – wait longer for help in their daily lives than do unattached older men (Gustafsson and Szebehely 2001).

None of the women in the study received any economic compensation when caring for ailing husbands. One of them instead found herself in a financial predicament when her husband, after many years of home care, was moved to a care facility and most of his pension went to covering the cost. Consequently her standard of living decreased, leading to money worries and social isolation. Many women in Sweden today have similar experiences. They have done what was expected of them, but without this work being assigned a value that entitles them to security in old age.

Housework and time

The unseen portion of women's work in the home has made it difficult to measure it in time management studies. Attempts have nevertheless been made, the first in the 1930s, when the purpose was in part to raise the status of housework and in part to provide suggestions for improvements that would lighten the workload. In this and subsequent studies it became evident that across the entire social spectrum, wives of small farmers had the heaviest work burden, even compared to men (Boalt 1983).

An effort was made to find measurement techniques that accurately reflected women's daily lives. In addition to calculating work time in hours and minutes, there was an attempt at a qualitative assessment, for instance to establish the work pace by studying how many times a day women working in the home shifted from one task to another. The average for women with children was 80 times, but figures of up to 140 were recorded. These results are most likely applicable today as well and reveal a work situation that demands great flexibility, with many tasks performed simultaneously.

The home itself and the way it accommodated the activities of mother and children was also a topic of interest. Was there enough space for children to play indoors? Was there enough space for a baby carriage in the apartment or by the stairs? Were the stairs steep? How was the entryway configured? Many women in our study pointed out how important it was that they could keep an eye on the children while going about their own work, not least when the children were playing outdoors.

Since men were not expected to be involved in housework during this period, their possible contribution was not investigated. In the 1960s and '70s, when public debate about gender equality accelerated in Sweden, studies also began measuring the time men devoted to household tasks, focusing primarily on the differences between the way men's and women's time was apportioned. There have not, however, been any new attempts to reflect the qualitative aspects or pace of the work.

Clock time and process time

The methods used in modern time management studies were originally developed to meet the needs of industry by focusing on how long it took to perform specific tasks. The sociologist Karen Davies called this clock time and questioned whether it can be used to measure work in the home, in particular caregiving, which is largely task- and need-driven and consequently can neither be predicted nor assigned a time duration in advance. There is no way to know, for instance, when a child will need comforting and how long this will take, or in which situations children will require attention or intervention. This type of work must be allowed to take whatever time is needed, which Davies called process time (Davies 1987, 1990).

This brings us back to the question of how unseen aspects of work can be measured and assessed. Time management studies done in Sweden in recent decades (the latest in 2010-11), calculating how people apportion their time in daily life, do not attempt to do so. To summarize, they demonstrate that for men and women between the ages of 20 and 64 the total work time per week is about the same, 50-60 hours. Men's work in the home and women's work at salaried jobs have both increased, but men continue to work more hours outside the home while women devote more of their time to housework. After deducting time for personal needs (sleep, eating, personal hygiene), the available "free time" is approximately the same for women and men, 33 and 35 hours per week respectively.

In these studies, time devoted to salaried work was equated with the number of hours *present* at the workplace, regardless of whether actual work was performed. In the private sphere, however, only the clock time for specific activities was measured, for instance how long it took to do the dishes or feed a child. In other words, the underlying assumptions differ for measurements of paid and unpaid work, and consequently they cannot be compared. The time required for taking responsibility for others, for being present and paying attention but without performing clearly defined tasks measurable in clock time, is not accounted for in the domestic sphere. Studies since the early 1990s nevertheless demonstrate that women do housework and spend their "free time" with children around them to a significantly greater degree than men do (Statistics Sweden 1990/1991, 2000/2001 and 2010/2011).

Free and restricted time

Women in this study revealed the actual extent of work time in the home, with the constraints on time and mobility that caregiving responsibilities entailed. In most families with children, the husband and father felt free to leave the house whenever he pleased under the assumption that his wife would be responsible for the children. The women, in contrast, almost always had to negotiate free time with their husbands. The entire time they were at home they were "on call" and expected to be available and aware of others' needs, those of children, husbands, whether healthy or ailing, and other relatives.

Thus actual free time was, and remains, significantly less than the statistics in time management studies indicate. We define "free time" as applying solely in the absence of responsibility for others, with no obstacles to leaving the house or pursuing personal interests without being disturbed. Only if free time is seen this way can caregiving responsibility in the private sphere be compared to analogous paid work, for instance as a childcare provider or healthcare professional.

Studies that cite averages also disguise the fact that the intensity of work varies over time and among individuals. A number of women in our study described periods in their lives when they worked virtually around the clock, primarily during the years when children lived at home or when ailing relatives required care. Wives of farmers described intense workdays determined by the season, during which they had virtually no time to themselves. Work was also tied to various calendar dates: holidays, among which Christmas was particularly mentioned, birthdays, and so on. Some women found the extra labor connected with these events extremely stressful. There is reason to believe that these "work peaks" routinely affect women more than men, even in younger generations. In studies that focus solely on the ordinary workweek this additional burden remains unseen.

Older people's time

Work after the usual age of retirement also goes unnoticed in time management studies, including Swedish ones. Some women we interviewed continued to care for healthy husbands in old age, sometimes putting more effort into this over time. One third of them assumed the additional time-consuming work of caring for ailing husbands. Many also devoted time and attention to helping their adult children and taking care of grandchildren. We view it as disturbing and an insult to the older segment of the population that modern time management studies have taken no notice of this contribution. The importance of caregiving in the private sphere for social welfare and the national economy remains unseen as a result.

Unpaid work and health

Despite the burden that responsibility for home and family entailed, many of the women saw this as the most significant contribution they had made. For women with children, knowing that they had provided security and a good home contributed to a sense of wellbeing even in old age, bringing out feelings of pleasure and pride when they looked back on their working lives. On an everyday basis, work in the home could offer greater self-determination than did salaried work. It also encompassed experiences of aesthetic pleasure and gratification.

At the same time, many women described symptoms that they connected with their responsibility for the family. These included fatigue, feelings of guilt and inadequacy, worry, stress and isolation. Physically demanding tasks and repetitive motion or uncomfortable posture caused strain. Among women who had cared for an ailing husband or a child day and night for many years, several had fallen or experienced ongoing pain in arms, neck or back from this work. This drew our attention to the work-related injuries that may occur in connection with household chores or caregiving in the private sphere. Accidents in the home, however, are categorized as occurring during "free time" in Sweden and have never been encompassed by protective legislation or insurance policies for work-related injury. A risk of chemical injury also exists, not least in the form of over-sensitivity and hand eczema.

Summary

That women were responsible for family life and the home was an explicit norm when participants in the study were young. Despite progress toward equality, in contemporary Sweden this total responsibility continues, in heterosexual families, to fall primarily on women. Many of the tasks and skills required are not identified in studies of housework and childcare, including time management studies, and consequently they are rendered unseen as work. Such tasks include organizing and planning, being physically present, and being aware of and responsive to the needs of family members. Then as now, the family's economic situation affects the extent and burden of work in the home and consequently the stress and worry associated with it.

The unreciprocated services that most of the married women in the study provided their husbands meant that in practice they served as their husbands' housekeepers. Their stories revealed that a central question relating to working conditions in the home and their impact on health was the degree to which husbands respected their wives' work and helped make it less taxing. With this in mind, we believe that women living in heterosexual relationships who are assigned or take on primary responsibility for children and the home will continue to be dependent on their husbands' attitudes and actions, thus giving men a major influence on women's domestic work environment.

11

Paid Work

The time spent in the work force varied among participants in the study, with the greatest differences between unmarried and married women. Single women worked for pay and were self-supporting most of their adult lives, two of them also supporting families, while nearly all the married women were at least periodically financially dependent on their husbands. The husbands' preferences strongly influenced whether or not they worked outside the home. Those wanting to be in the work force might also be hindered by the lack of available jobs or access to childcare.

Some women, primarily those with a higher education, had the opportunity to choose their professions. Those without much formal education were often forced to take whatever jobs they could find locally, in industry or in the caregiving or household sectors.

Health benefits

Whether or not they had chosen their line of work themselves, almost all the women described positive experiences in the work force. During the period that encompassed their working lives it was often assumed, however, that gainful employment was not as meaningful to women, especially married women, as to men. In research, paid employment has long been treated as giving women a new role in addition to their traditional ones of wife and mother (cf. Artazcoz et al. 2004). The question has been raised as to whether such engagement is beneficial or harmful to women's health. Multiple role theories and concepts such as role overload, role conflict and role enhancement have been used as analysis tools (see Forssén and Carlstedt 2007; compare Waldron et al. 1998). When, on the other hand, women's own experiences have been taken into account, paid work is highlighted as both desired and appreciated, irrespective of marital status and limits set by social norms, rules and legislation. Such research has established that employed women, regardless of education and marital status, were more satisfied than full-time housewives. Women in low status jobs who were assumed to work principally out of economic necessity also regarded their jobs, rather than their home and family obligations, as the main source of feelings of usefulness and importance (Ferree 1976; compare Artazcoz et al. 2004; Roos et al. 2005).

In accordance with other research findings, our study shows that employment promotes women's wellbeing by offering increased self-esteem, life satisfaction, social contacts outside the family, financial independence and a work identity (Sorensen and Verbrugge 1987; Repetti et al 1989). Since money is a strong measure of social worth, having an income of their own also strengthened the women's position in relation to their husbands and helped redress existing inequalities (compare Ross and Mirowsky 1995). This factor contributed to the secondary school teacher's satisfaction about earning the same salary as her husband. For women married to anti-social or dominating men, the possibility of leaving the house and meeting other people in a paid job was particularly important.

Thus, among the health-promoting effects of paid work for both women and men, some factors related to gender and power, such as having a personal income and using paid employment as "a room of one's own," stand out as especially significant for women, irrespective of social class and family constellation (Ross and Mirowsky 1995; Hemström 2005; Håkansson et el. 2005). There is also strong evidence that unemployment is particularly disadvantageous to women's health, quite apart from loss of income (Ross and Mirowsky 1995; Walters 2004; Roos et al. 2005).

Through their paid work, some participants in our study were able to manage and even alleviate pain and illness. Feeling needed, having control over their work, receiving acknowledgment, having fun, and establishing a structure for the day were explanations they gave for such health benefits and their willingness to work through illness. This is in line with the suggestion that a job may be valuable by promoting "perceived health," while not always improving "physical functioning" (Ross and Mirowsky 1995).

In sum, we regard the question of whether work outside the home is beneficial or harmful to women's health as improperly formulated. It does not take into account women's own wishes and statements and ignores salaried employment and an income of one's own as women's indisputable right. The question also overlooks the significant number of women who have always worked for pay without being registered in the statistics as members of the labor force. Further, it ignores the fact, evident in the following section in this chapter, that women's work-related health and illness above all depend on their working conditions.[6]

Low status, low pay, and segregation

In spite of their positive experiences in the work force, nearly all of the women gave examples of ways in which they were particularly exposed because they were women, one of them also as an immigrant. This was especially true for those working in typically female occupations with low wages and few opportunities for advancement. Many found their work environments unpleasant and had memories of being poorly treated. To some degree this was also the case for those who held relatively high positions in male-dominated professions, the engineer and the physician. They sometimes perceived themselves as having lower status than male colleagues in the work group and might be treated differently because they were women. The only two who did not describe negative experiences related to gender were the secondary school teacher and the artist, the latter with some reservations, since she did not have a high public profile.

Concerning women's low wages, we have already noted that in the 1930s the social activist Alva Myrdal drew attention to the tradition of equating poorly paid work with women's work (see Chapter 6). One way of maintaining unequal wage scales was to keep men and women in separate sectors of the labor market: "When employers were unable or unwilling to raise women's wages, it became all the more important to decide what should be considered men's and women's work assignments." Myrdal goes on to describe contracts that included unmotivated specification of the segments of various tasks that should be performed by women versus men (Myrdal 1938: 32-33). Her piercing analysis received little attention, however, and it was not until the 1970s that concepts such as gender segregation in the workplace and the power relationship between women and men came under discussion, in the women's movement and in feminist scholarship. As we see it, the gender theory that was introduced in Sweden at that time (Hirdman 1990), based on gender distinctions

---

6 For a more detailed description and discussion of health-promoting aspects of a paid job, as well as further references, see Forssén and Carlstedt 2007.

and the primacy of the male norm,[7] is a latter-day extension of Alva Myrdal's ideas.

That criteria for classifying some work tasks as "for women" and others "for men" had more to do with the status of the work than physical requirements or technical expertise was emphasized in a government inquiry initiated and led by female contemporaries of Myrdal (SOU 1938: 47). Industries such as textiles and shoe manufacturing that employed two study participants were included in the inquiry as examples of low-paying sectors dominated by women. Study participants also described physically demanding work as cleaners and in industrial kitchens, likewise considered female occupations. Common to all these jobs was that they offered few career opportunities; foremen were almost invariably men.

Even in white-collar jobs, opportunities for advancement were more tied to gender than to education and experience. The telegraph operator in our study experienced this; her lower position as a woman gave her less possibility of promotion and a salary raise than men in the same workplace, despite having better qualifications. An analogous unequal relationship pertained between typists, a female-dominated occupation, and typographers, who were mostly men. Both jobs demanded precision and speed, but typographers had higher status and higher salaries (Humlesjö 1999).

Perceptions about which types of work are appropriate for each sex have continuously changed as the labor market itself has evolved; some sectors have disappeared while new ones have emerged. The introduction of new machines has generally raised the status and pay scales of a job and usually led to a higher percentage of men in that occupation (Humlesjö 1999).

Bodily contact

Occupations that include caregiving and household chores have remained poorly paid women's work with low status. To understand why, we can refer once again to the concepts of "nurturing" and "home-nurturing" and the way women traditionally have been expected to take on these tasks. When the public sector that includes many such jobs was expanded in the 1960s, formal training was seldom necessary, which in turn was

---

[7] The primacy of the male norm may be defined as a general acceptance of men's rights taking precedence and men having the highest status in society.

used as a motive for the low pay scale.[8] That this work involves care of the body has also been a factor in the meager wages; the closer the proximity to dirt and bodily excretions, the lower the status of the work.[9] House cleaning and laundry can likewise be associated with maintaining bodily cleanliness. According to this argument, women's work removing other people's dirt and grime contributes to their low social status.

The low status, past and present, of cleaning associated with bodily functions became apparent when research was presented in Sweden on the way toilets were constructed and the impact this had on those who cleaned them (Linn 1985). The investigation attracted a great deal of attention, but public debate focused less on the quality and significance of the research than on whether it was "acceptable" to do research on this topic. The dissertation was mocked in the media, yet another example of trivializing the work of cleaning up after others.

In agriculture as well, the division of labor was associated with the body. The connection between milking and "nurturing" and the intimate physical contact with animal bodies that milking by hand entailed no doubt played a role in making this a woman's job. When technology transformed the work, bodily contact with the animals was reduced and milking became a task for both men and women (see Sommestad 1992).

Relational work

Study participants employed in caregiving professions were expected to be empathetic and able to build relations. Simultaneously they often had little control over their work situation and decisions affecting patients. Difficult "caught-in-the-middle" situations arose when sensitivity to the needs of those in their care had to be combined with the necessity of meeting the demands of superiors: they had great responsibility but little power. The work situation remains the same today in these occupations as well as in teaching, social work, and other female-dominated fields (Järvholm and Reutervall 2012). For women in many other occupations as well, concern for others and building relationships is often a significant aspect of work. In our study the engineer and the grocery shop clerk dealt with relationship

---

8 The low pay scale remains in effect, despite the fact that almost all occupations require at least a secondary school education today.
9 The exceptions are certain professions calling for close bodily contact that have higher status because they require scientific knowledge. One example is medicine.

issues and listened to confidences that had nothing to do with their actual work assignments.

The continuous physical and emotional attention required by relational work and responsibility for others can make the work exhausting. Time for this type of interpersonal interaction can only rarely be set aside during regular work hours, leading to time pressure and unpaid overtime. Stress, worry, and guilt feelings about not doing a good job are consequences. Since relational work sometimes encompasses potentially volatile individuals, for instance when caring for psychiatric patients or those suffering from dementia, it requires both emotional and physical preparedness for violence, which women are twice as likely as men to encounter on the job.

The skills called for in relational work are generally unseen and seldom mentioned in job descriptions. This "silent expertise" is difficult to put into words, not least for those who put it into practice, and is not always perceived as a skill or qualification. It rarely plays a significant role in promoting women's careers, nor does it lead to salary increases. When such expertise is neither valued nor brought to light, it can also be called "silenced expertise."

It appears that women in all occupations are expected to have competence in and to carry out certain practical and nurturing tasks. In our study, for instance, the secretary related that she considered it "natural" that she help her male boss with personal as well as professional matters. The physician, on the other hand, found that female staff members did not assist her the same way they did male physicians; instead she was expected to manage most aspects of patient care herself (compare Davies 2001). As a result the work situation is different for women and men, even within the same profession. That many women in lower positions willingly take on service tasks in the workplace may be motivated by their wish to be accepted and appreciated. This is especially true if career opportunities in other ways are limited.

Sexual harassment

The women in this study have contributed to our awareness that sexual vulnerability in the workplace is not a new phenomenon. About half the women experienced some form of harassment that frightened and humiliated them, though several did protest. It is difficult to determine what effect these affronts, verbal and physical, had on them in the long run. It was nevertheless clear that they were among the most painful memories from their working lives.

In recent years, "sexual harassment" has become the accepted term for sexually based affronts, and the prevalence of the phenomenon has received public attention, in Sweden and globally (JämO 2007; Wong 2010). It is classified as a work environment issue and a widespread health problem and occurs in all sectors of the educational system and labor market, migrants and women of color being particularly exposed. The number of unreported cases remains high. The feelings of shame that are closely associated with all forms of sexualized violence, and fear of losing a job, are reasons women do not dare report what has occurred. Female students may put up with harassment for fear that otherwise their future opportunities will be jeopardized (Högskoleverket 2000). The harassment of schoolgirls has only in recent years attracted attention (Witkowska 2005). We know that overall, sexual harassment undercuts the victim's sense of control and self-determination.

Issues concerning HBTQ (homosexual, bisexual, transgender, and queer) individuals were not openly discussed during much of the lifetimes of women in the study. As noted previously, homosexual acts were criminalized until the mid-1940s and after that, until the 1970s, homosexuality was classified as an illness. Many HBTQ individuals in this generation were forced to hide their orientation to enter the labor market and retain a position there. In Sweden today, the medical profession and political powers-that-be have affirmed that homosexuality is a sexual orientation among others. Those who do not conform to the perceived heterosexual norm nevertheless continue to encounter prejudice and disparagement.

Improved rights – but lack of parity

One significant difference between present-day Sweden and the period when the women in this study were young is that the norm of the stay-at-home housewife has been replaced by the expectation that all women will support themselves. The understanding that women and men should have equal opportunities in the labor market has both political and popular support. Legal reforms pertaining to the labor market and family circumstances as well as access to childcare have promoted this goal. In addition, more women than men today have professional training and quite a few acquire a higher education, even in fields earlier dominated by men. An increasing number of women also reach higher positions, although a smaller percent than among men with the same education. Women continue, on the average, to earn less than men, even when they have the same education and job assignments.

It is thus apparent that unequal conditions between the sexes still pertain in the labor market. Many women also continue to choose, or be steered into, fields that are designated as particularly appropriate for them. Even while growing up, girls are prompted in that direction; the gendered division of responsibility that they observe and live with also has an impact. Research on the inherent capabilities of girls versus boys, which is increasingly in demand, may also be used to support traditional choices. Although differences between women and men, if they exist at all, are significantly less than differences within each sex – the latter often related to class – data that support differences between the sexes often weigh heavily, for instance in advising young people about what occupation to choose (see Fausto-Sterling 2011).

Single-sex workplaces thus remain common for both women and men.[10] A majority of women are employed in low-paying, low-status occupations with limited opportunities for advancement, in caregiving, cleaning, retail, kitchen work and industry. These are fields in which heavy lifting, monotonous tasks, uncomfortable work posture, high demands under time pressure and lack of autonomy are widespread. Such pressing situations, or "job strain," lead to an increased risk of illness (Karasek and Theorell 1990). These factors that jeopardize health have not improved in recent years; in fact, there are signs that the situation is becoming worse, particularly regarding stress at work (Järvholm and Reutervall 2012). Statistics show that women have more sleep disturbances due to job pressure, are more frequently physically exhausted after work, and are more likely than men to feel they have too much to do (Statistics Sweden 2012a).

In workplaces where both women and men are employed, they are often assigned different work tasks, where men's assignments continue to be seen as more demanding or qualified and as a consequence are more highly valued than women's. In reality, women's tasks are often just as strenuous and demanding and require just as much competence with respect to technical skills, planning and organization (Elwér 2013).[11]

---

10 In 2008, a comparison between female-dominated and male-dominated sectors demonstrated, for instance, that the average salary for a full-time construction worker was SEK 26,400 per month, while the corresponding figure for a practical nurse was SEK 18,500. Both occupations require a secondary school degree but are strongly male and female dominated respectively.

11 In recent years issues connected with the evaluation of women's and men's work have attracted growing attention, in some instances due to lawsuits in the Swedish Labour Court. For instance, midwifery, an increasingly technical profession, has been compared to the better-paid, male-dominated occupation of hospital technician – albeit to date without improving the circumstances of midwives.

Moreover, tools adapted to the male body are taxing for women to handle, and protective equipment designed for men may not fit women properly. Taken together, these divergent working conditions for women and men lead to different injuries and illnesses and help explain, for instance, why women experience more muscle pain than men (Messing 1998; Vingård and Kilhlbom 2001; Lewis and Mathiasen 2013).

A further problem, especially in the caregiving fields, is that employers often offer only part-time work or positions in which work is divided into split shifts spread out over the day, sometimes in different places with long commutes between them (Mårtensson and Yeshimock 2013). When workdays are extended and schedules are erratic, stress, worry, fatigue and problems arranging childcare are likely to arise.

The labor market has also become less stable, especially for women, with a growing tendency to replace regular positions with short-term contractual ones. Many women circulate among different segments of the labor market: regular salaried employment alternates with education and training, substitute positions, parental leave, and periods of unemployment. These factors contribute to making present-day women, like women of previous generations, society's reserve work force or buffer – despite the fact that women are more likely than men to have a higher education (Statistics Sweden 2012b). There also continue to be major differences among women with regard to work environment and circumstances. In Sweden, conditions for migrant women, with or without documents, are often the worst (Gavana 2010; Bohlin 2012). We wonder what opportunities women in exposed positions in the labor market have to find jobs that do not jeopardize their health? What hope can they have of maintaining health in the work environments open to them?

Sick leave

When the women in this study entered the work force there was no universal health insurance in Sweden, so they often worked despite being ill; staying home meant no income for days missed. After the universal health insurance law was enacted in 1955 several of them, primarily those with little education and strenuous jobs, were on sick leave for shorter or longer periods later in life. Some had taken early retirement when they became seriously ill or no longer had the stamina to continue.

The health insurance law includes compensation for income lost due to illness.[12] Among both men and women of working age, the percentage on sick leave is, and always has been, significantly higher for those with little education (Rostila and Toivanen 2012; Hensing 2012). The largest number of long-term sick leaves and early retirements are found in fields where women are the majority, and women are on sick leave approximately twice as often as men (Hensing 2012). Psychological and musculoskeletal conditions are the most common reasons, the former increasing more than any other cause today (Försäkringskassan 2013). Women in higher positions are also more sick-listed than men of similar rank. In social debate these gender differences have been presented as difficult to account for. As we see it, unequal conditions in the working lives of women and men, as described above, explain much of the disparity.

Work-related injuries

The current law on work-related injuries went into effect in 1976. At that time the oldest women in this study were reaching retirement age. Several of them had suffered injuries that in the 1990s, during a brief period when the law was generously applied, might have been classified as work-related. Before and after that time, however, the Social Insurance Agency's narrow interpretation of the law has resulted in the approval of far fewer claims of work-related injury in female-dominated sectors than in male-dominated ones. The reason, according to the Agency's own analysts, is that research on such injuries has focused primarily on fields dominated by men, which has provided more scientific evidence of the kind required for approval. Research has, for instance, examined isolated accident cases rather than injuries caused by stationary posture on the job, repetitive motion, or prolonged emotional and physical stress (Vingård and Kihlbom 2001; Mattsson 2011; Arbetsskadekommissionen 2012). Few claims are filed related to healthcare or social welfare jobs despite the fact that injuries caused by heavy lifting and violent patients and clients are common. Furthermore, follow-up investigations are more thorough for men than for women, and for professions with higher salary levels where more

---

12 The Swedish Social Insurance Agency is responsible for its implementation. Sick leave longer than one week requires a doctor's certificate describing the effect of the ailment on work capabilities, but Agency staff always make the final decision about whether compensation will be paid. Beginning some years ago, the first two weeks of sick pay have been covered by the employer.

men are employed. When investigating claims of work-related injury, women's personal sphere is examined to a greater degree than is the case for men and may be cited as a "competing activity" to motivate denying the claim (Mattsson 2011: 36). Women are thus caught between conflicting demands: when injured in connection with work, their expected responsibility for home and care of the family is held against them.

Paid work and time

Those of our participants who had children and had been gainfully employed described, as a consequence of the total workload, an almost constant feeling of being pressed for time. They wanted fewer working hours, both paid and unpaid. However, few of them could afford to reduce their paid work time, especially if they were single mothers, and moreover part-time work was less available than it is today. The result was that positive feelings about jobs were often obscured by guilt for not satisfying the norm of being stay-at-home mothers and the fear of damaging their children by their absence. The lack of daycare facilities (still the case in most European countries outside Scandinavia) also made the women worry about the children while at work. Study participants confirmed what social activist Alva Myrdal emphasized in the 1930s: the problem was not women working outside the home, but that society was not organized to enable women with salaried employment to be mothers (Myrdal 1938). During the working lives of women in the study very little changed in this regard. Since then there have been extensive changes in Swedish society to help make it possibile for parents to combine salaried employment and family responsibilities. From the 1960s and onwards, the length of paid maternity leave has successively increased, and in the 1970s parental leave was introduced, giving parents the right to divide the leave time between them. Since the early 2000s parents in Sweden are entitled to a total of 15 months of paid leave in connection with the birth of a child, with economic compensation based on salary. Except in unusual circumstances, the father is legally obliged to take at least 60 days of parental leave. There is ongoing political debate about increasing the leave period and introducing a requirement that it be more evenly divided between parents, which is seen as a step to promote equality; in 2012, 80 percent of leave time was used by women. Many influential politicians and several major political parties are nevertheless opposed, with the argument that families themselves should decide how leave time is shared.

In the 1970s the system of daycare centers was also greatly expanded in Sweden. Today all children of working parents, or parents who are looking for work, have the right to publicly financed childcare from the age of one.

Since part-time employment was seldom available to women in our study, working outside the regular labor market might provide an alternative that enabled them to manage childcare responsibilities. Today, parents of children up to the age of eight have the legal right to reduce their work time to 75 percent of a full-time 40-hour week. However, only women who can afford a reduced income, in practice those living with partners or who themselves are highly paid, have the freedom to choose reduced work time. This eliminates the large group of low-income single mothers, who furthermore often have the longest and most strenuous workdays, including both paid and unpaid work, and no one to share household and caring tasks.

Among married or cohabiting couples the possibility of reducing work time is more often utilized by women than by men. Although some men do reduce their work hours, they are so few that they are scarcely discernible statistically and, as a group, fathers of small children are among those who work the most hours outside the home. Even in their free time, fathers spend more time outside the home than mothers do. In addition, more mothers than fathers make use of the right to stay home caring for ill children, with compensation from the Social Insurance Agency. The problem of absent fathers that many women in the study described thus remains for many women in contemporary Sweden (Harrysson 2012; Statistics Sweden 2003, 2012). Furthermore, both pregnancy and the care of small children are difficult to combine with present-day conditions in many sectors of the labor market, including split schedules, demands for overtime work or being available outside regular work hours. As long as work in the private sphere is not equally shared, combining full-time salaried employment with raising children will continue to be a greater problem for women than for men.

Since the mid-1980s, proposals for reduced work hours for everyone have been under political discussion in Sweden. The larger parties have always rejected this reform, claiming it would harm the national economy. For many women, a reduction in the number of work hours considered "normal" would nevertheless have major health benefits – providing this did not entail a reduction in salary. Most likely men's health and quality of life would also benefit from spending more time in the home (Harryson 2012). In addition, an across-the-board reduction in salaried work would give people's daily needs in the private sphere, both emotional and practical, increased status in relation to the demands of work outside the home.

Career and power within the family

That far more women than men reduce their work time can be explained by economic factors. Since men often earn higher salaries than women, the most advantageous choice financially for most families, at least in the short run, is that the woman reduces her work hours. A contributing factor is that in most families women still have the responsibility of seeing to it that the work gets done in the home (see Chapter 10). Another, less obvious motive might be that this choice maintains the man's higher status, socially as well as in the relationship, which he, and sometimes his female partner, finds comfortable. In families where the husband is on a fast career track, the woman's support by taking on much of the household work can be a way of demonstrating her love and ensuring that she will be loved in return (Jonasdottir 1991; Magnusson 2008). This is especially likely if the woman's own career opportunities are limited.

Women sometimes try to make their outside employment invisible at home, adapting to a "marriage contract" where a woman's worth and foundation for being loved is based on her performance as (house)wife and caregiver and threatened by engagement and success outside the home. In our study, even highly educated married women made accommodations to avoid marital discord. By not pursuing further training in their fields, both the secondary school teacher and the physician circumvented further rivalry with their husbands, who worked in the same profession. When women make such adaptations they reduce their own opportunities for advancement in the work force and the social benefits that accompany it, both in the short term and over time. The current pension system, based on lifetime earnings, works against women who eschew professional advancement in favor of their husbands. Economic advantages and better career opportunities thus enable men to maintain their power over women, both privately and in the public sphere.

Approaching retirement

The final years in the work force varied among women in this study. Most of them wanted to stay in their jobs until retirement age. Some who had strenuous jobs but were given less demanding tasks toward the end managed to continue working longer than they could have done otherwise. One woman, the shop assistant, even chose to work long after the usual retirement age because she enjoyed her job so much. A study from this period showed that "elderly" (age 57 on average) female industrial workers were "less likely to be positively oriented towards retirement than were men" (Jacobson 1974). Although the reasons for this difference between the sexes were not explored, we speculate, drawing on comments of study participants, that a significant factor was women's greater need for "a room of their own," especially if their husbands had already retired. Those of our participants who were forced into early retirement, whether because of illness or organizational changes in the work place, described how much they missed their jobs and daily contact with their co-workers. Others, worn out by their work, were satisfied and felt a sense of release when they were able to retire.

Today there are large groups of older women, particularly in retail, hotel and restaurant work, in caregiving professions and in industry, who run the risk of being trapped in physically and psychologically strenuous jobs as long as they remain in the work force. The nature of the work often makes it impossible to improve conditions significantly. This prompts the question of how to design work environments so that employees of all ages can stay healthy and continue to work productively, and to find ways to take advantage of and pass along the acquired expertise of older workers.

Summary

The rights of women in the labor market have in many ways improved compared to previous generations. Few Swedish women today desire to work solely in the home, nor would this be economically feasible. In our study paid work was experienced as health-promoting through providing meaning, self-esteem, social relations, and a basis for self-determination and economic independence. Furthermore, it offered the women freedom from constant availability to the needs of their families and strengthened them in unequal or even abusive partner relationships. Distraction from pain and chronic ailments was another health-promoting aspect of employment.

Injustices and unequal circumstances between women and men were nevertheless a common thread in study participants' narratives of their working lives. Taking into consideration both positive and negative factors in women's working conditions, we once again assert that the frequently asked question as to whether gainful employment is beneficial or harmful to women's health is improperly framed. In line with our findings as well as with previous research, we consider it more important to investigate what leads to health and what causes illness in women's paid, private and combined workload.

12

Illness, Medical Care, and Society

Public healthcare

Beginning in the 1950s, the publicly financed healthcare system underwent significant expansion in Sweden. Everyone was to have equal access to medical treatment, regardless of income. Focus was primarily on specialized care according to the principle of separate clinics for each body part. Consequently individuals whose symptoms derived from long-term physical, social, or psychological strain, like many women in our study, or with complex or multiple illnesses could be misdiagnosed or overlooked. Expansion of primary care during the 1970s and '80s was intended to facilitate a more coherent approach to treatment, but since that time financial resources have once again been earmarked mainly for specialized clinics. Beginning in the 1990s, a private healthcare system has also evolved, though it, too, is mostly publicly financed and the cost to individual patients is low.

When the women in our study sought medical attention they usually encountered male physicians. Women in Sweden gained the right to pursue university studies in 1873 and the first female physician received her degree in 1888. It was not until 1923, however, that women doctors were allowed to work in the public sector, for instance at hospitals. During the 1930s and '40s, women constituted about 5 percent of the total number of physicians; by 1960 the figure had risen to approximately 20 percent. Thereafter came a sharp increase and at present women comprise a small majority of those completing medical school. Of doctors currently practicing, men nevertheless remain in the majority, as they do in administrative and policy-making positions in medical care, teaching, and research. The number of women and men is unevenly divided among various specialties. Gender-based discrimination with regard to salary and career opportunities continues to create gender inequality in the profession, as does sexual harassment.

(Ström 2014; Spak and Ålebring 2014).[13] Unequal opportunities also pertain in medical research.[14]

The first female physicians often focused specifically on women's health issues. They promoted women's right to have control over their bodies and their sexuality and drew attention to the connection between the economic difficulties many women faced and their poor health (Widerström 1924). Later in the twentieth century it was primarily female physicians who pointed out the ways male subjectivity had affected medical research and practice, and they continue to be far more likely to prioritize and investigate gender issues in medicine (Risberg et al. 2003; Risberg 2004). One explanation is that the experiences of many women doctors differ from those of male colleagues but are shared by most women, for instance concerning various kinds of discrimination and the risk of sexually based violence. Their situation as women has thus affected their stance on medical issues, just as is the case for men, but as a more deliberate choice. At the same time women's life experiences vary widely, and women doctors should not necessarily be expected to bring divergent or pioneering perspectives to their work.

The medicalization of female biology

In medicine, worldwide and for centuries a male-dominated profession, women's physical as well as mental illnesses have to a large extent been seen as correlated to their reproductive biology (Haraway 1991; Johannisson 2001). An underlying assumption is that the cyclical changes in the female body are something negative, a hindrance in life and work and not "normal." This has been applied to women's lives from puberty until old age, but from the 1960s until the late twentieth century, menopause was particularly in focus. The physical changes around age 50 that lead to the loss of childbearing capability were put forward as the beginning of a life-long condition of deficiency. Healthy women around the world were given hormone replacement therapy even if they did not suffer any uncomfortable symptoms in connection with menopause. Citing flawed research, medical experts asserted that this

---

13 This applies not only in Sweden but also internationally (Hinze 2004; Allen 2005; Riska 2011).

14 An attention-grabbing article in *Nature* established that to receive funding from the Swedish Medical Research Council (now the Swedish Research Council), women needed to be more than twice as qualified as men (Wennerås and Wold 1997).

treatment would keep women both young and healthy (see McPherson and Hemminki 2004). These recommendations remained in place until the early 2000s, when carefully controlled research revealed the high number of diseases and deaths linked to the treatment, particularly from breast cancer and thrombosis (Roousouw et al. 2002; Beral et al. 2003; Main et al. 2013).

Women in our study did not mention major problems at menopause. In spite of this some of them received extensive hormone treatment, and one had undergone a complete hysterectomy without understanding why. Over the course of several years, one participant had been prescribed estrogen for conditions as varied as a defective heart valve and pain in an arm, the latter a work-related injury. This delayed proper treatment and caused bleeding, pain, and the risk of other health problems before the correct diagnosis was made. Her experience illustrates the way even serious illnesses and injuries risk being overlooked when doctors interpret a woman's symptoms as menopause-related.

Feelings of shame associated with aging and loss of fertility may easily arise when experts focus on the natural aging process as a defect. Promotional material to Swedish physicians during these years advocated hormone treatment, arguing that this would enable women past childbearing age to retain their "femininity" and help doctors deal with "change-of-life females"[15](*Läkartidningen* 1993, 90: 88). Furthermore, when women are put on medication in response to normal biological processes they are transformed into patients without being ill. Such medicalization reinforces a negative perception of women's bodies and women's weaker position in society compared to men.

At present the days before the menstrual period begins are receiving a great deal of attention in the western world and what used to be treated as a variety of symptoms (premenstrual syndrome/PMS) has recently, in severe cases, been classified as a disorder, premenstrual dysphoric disorder (PMDD).[16] The disorder is assumed to have grave consequences for family and work life, and antidepressants are the current recommended treatment (Callaghan et al. 2008; Pilver et al.

---

15 The Swedish word "klimakterietant" has a distinctly condescending flavor implying that such women are overwrought.
16 In the *Diagnostic and Statistical Manual of Mental Disorders* (DSM), premenstrual dysphoric disorder (PMDD) has been moved from Appendix B (research diagnosis) in DSM-4 to the main body of DSM-5 (2012).

2011).[17] Unlike a simplistic biological explanation, research that takes into account women's personal history demonstrates that the symptoms are often connected to life circumstances and traumas (Studd and Nappi 2012). It has also been pointed out that PMS is absent in many non-western countries and that active management of symptoms by the women themselves can effectively reduce them (Ussher and Perz 2013). The perception that the female biological cycle is aberrant, an anomaly, has also motivated excluding women from pharmacological studies of drugs that they nevertheless are expected to take (Dresser 1993; Meinert 1995).

Women have, of course, advocated more research on female biology, but when medical science classifies normal processes as abnormal and biological factors are separated from the rest of life, the questions and interpretations become oversimplified, misdirected and frequently prejudicial. An alternative perspective would be to view the female cycle as normal and to draw attention to the proactive ways women may respond to it.

Pain and gender

From the 1950s on, all the women in our study had access to low-cost healthcare. Even so, many of them felt that they were not taken seriously, or even listened to at all, when they described their symptoms to the doctor. This was especially common when they sought help for back pain or pain in muscles and joints. The disparaging expression "throbbing-burning-pain biddy," referring to female patients with pain symptoms, was frequently used in healthcare during this time. The expression might even be entered in their medical records to discourage other physicians from paying "unnecessary attention" to their symptoms. Many women were also diagnosed with "psychological deficiencies" when they suffered from pain and fatigue. This happened, we know, to at least one participant in our study,[18] and we have periodically seen it ourselves in our work as medical doctors. Belittling terms like these demonstrate that women were generally regarded as complainers and as emotionally fragile

---

17 The pharmaceutical industry has strongly supported this approach, for instance in advertisements where texts like "My monthly mood swings take their toll/Bring discord, harm, and loss of control" are embroidered in beautiful cross-stitched designs (CNSpharma/H Lundbeck AB; Läkartidningen 2012).
18 We have had access to the women's medical records.

and nervous, and consequently their symptoms were dismissed as exaggerated or illusory. No equivalent condescending appellations have ever been assigned to men.

Women in our study, on the other hand, blamed many of their symptoms on strenuous work, whether paid, unpaid or taken together. Among them were the cleaner who had to haul many pails of water up and down "endless" flights of stairs, the cleaner at construction sites, and those who worked in factories. Domestic chores had often been strenuous as well; several participants had carried out this work since childhood.

In Sweden, joint and muscle pain remains common among women over 45 and far more common among women than men (Statistics Sweden 2012b). Rheumatic illnesses are twice as frequent among women. Despite this, women with joint and muscle pain receive less attention in the healthcare system than do men with equivalent symptoms, and are more likely to be assigned nonspecific diagnoses and given mood-altering drugs as treatment (Hamberg et al. 2002; Hamberg 2008). This suggests that men's symptoms more often are seen as "real" while women's are attributed to psychological factors. One consequence of this approach is that underlying causes in women's work environments are not addressed. Furthermore, compared with men, women with joint and muscle problems have access to fewer and less costly rehabilitation efforts, whether through state-sponsored programs or their employers (Eklund 2010). These circumstances play a role in the frequent and lengthy periods of sick leave women with these diagnoses must take. The prolonged strain experienced by women living in abusive relationships also leads to pain (Hamberg et al. 1998; Wijma et al. 2007).

Cardiovascular disease

Four participants in this study had suffered heart attacks at a relatively young age, and in all cases the correct diagnosis was not made until long after symptoms became evident. Intense fatigue and chest or neck pain were early signs, but since the women were used to these symptoms they did not consider cardiovascular disease as a possible cause and instead kept on working as usual as long as they could. One of them, however, did suspect heart problems, but staff at the local clinic refused to examine her.

The reason the women did not take their symptoms seriously was probably that cardiovascular diseases, in particular heart attacks, were associated with men – by medical science and consequently by the general population – despite the fact that these are the most common causes of death in both sexes. For many years, research was conducted almost exclusively on male patients. Consequently women who had suffered a heart attack or were at risk for one might receive the wrong treatment or none at all; they were less likely, for example, to receive emergency or intensive care. Results from research on men were also automatically applied to women as well. More recently it has been established that changes in the blood vessels that cause angina may differ between women and men, a factor that must be taken into consideration when new patients are examined (Hamberg 2008). As is the case with muscular pain, in diagnosed cases of acute heart problems or stroke in Sweden, more resources are devoted to support and rehabilitation for men than for women (Smirthwaite 2007).

The women themselves had become aware later in life of the possible connection between their heart problems and their work circumstances, in salaried positions as well as in private life. The farm wife who had a heart attack when scarcely 50 described having more work than her physical strength could handle as well as little control over working hours. The physician in our study mentioned having no backup or support with childcare responsibilities and too many demands on the job, where as a female psychiatrist she encountered special expectations. The district nurse married to a minister had a heart attack shortly after her husband's retirement party, where her extensive efforts at his side went unnoticed. In her professional role she took care of battered women after the workday was over. Today, the type of stress these women described is seen as a major reason that the incidence of cardiovascular disease among women in the caregiving professions has not declined, as it has in other categories, but rather has risen (Bäckström and Wamala 2012; Järvholm and Reutervall 2012). This is also the case with regard to stroke. Among the women mentioned above, only the farm wife received confirmation from healthcare professionals of the connection between heart attack and a heavy workload.

Several of the women in unhappy marriages were constantly on edge due to their husbands' unpredictable temper and behavior. Research has demonstrated that for women, stress (anxiety, tension, fear) in the marital relationship is just as great a risk factor for heart attack and angina as stress at work. Marital stress also worsens the prognosis in affected women. Studies conducted on men do not reach the same conclusion (Orth-Gomér et al. 1997; 2000).

Mental health issues

Two study participants had been diagnosed with depression, followed by treatment in the form of medication or hospitalization. A significant factor in mastering the illness was their own ability to make changes in their work or life situations.

Throughout the western world, twice as many women as men are diagnosed with depression. Since significant gender differences manifest themselves at puberty, the rising levels of sex hormones, believed to lead to an innate fragility in female physiology, have often been held accountable (Kessler 2003). Less attention has been paid to the disparity in circumstances and expectations that boys and girls encounter as they approach adulthood (Hammarström et al. 2009) or women and men experience in adult life. In recent years, however, sexual bias in diagnosing depression has come under increasing scrutiny. Because diagnostic criteria were developed based on studies done exclusively on women, female patients run a greater risk of being over-diagnosed, while depression in men, with somewhat different symptoms, may be overlooked (Hirschbein 2006; Hamberg 2008). Symptoms of depression in women are strongly associated with negative conditions in the work place, lack of equality in the marital relationship, and financial difficulties (Hammarström and Phillips 2012). Antidepressants are prescribed more frequently to women with an abbreviated education living in poverty than to other groups (Statistics Sweden 2006).

Some women in the study had felt depressed and anxious in the months after giving birth, but none of them turned to the healthcare system for advice or treatment. One woman linked these feelings to a traumatic experience; another, who had no negative memories of labor and delivery, associated her anxiety and dejection with a sense of alienation in the marital relationship. Yet another had just lost her own mother, the only person who might have offered support in her new role. Medically, post-partum depression is regarded as a separate form of the illness, with hormone changes a significant cause, but the connection to socio-economic and psycho-social factors, including marital conflict and the partner's lack of support, has received increasing attention (O'Hara and McCabe 2013). Another underlying element may be previous experience of sexual abuse (Söderquist et al. 2009). Depression that develops in connection with childbirth can subsequently lead to decreased self-esteem, since women feel they have missed out on an important period in their lives and that their emotional distance may have harmed their children.

Health insurance and women's daily lives

Since salaried work, in particular that of men, has been the central focus of social organization and legislation, women's real-life situation has often been left aside. This becomes evident in connection with the universal health insurance law that was introduced in Sweden in 1955. Women who, in keeping with the norm of the period, were housewives, without an income of their own, were granted the right to a small "base sum" for sick leave. Application of this paragraph of the law was nevertheless problematic from the start, and it was believed necessary to establish rules regarding work in the home while on sick leave. For example, women were permitted to cook for themselves and the children, but not for their husbands. Those with memories from this time describe an ongoing conflict between what they were allowed to do and work they felt was necessary to accomplish, and constant fear that an inspector from the Social Insurance Agency would appear.[19]

This type of investigation of women on sick leave continued later in the century, most recently in the 1990s (see *Dagens Nyheter* 29 August 2006; 30 August 2006; 1 June 2008). At that time the Agency argued that women with a family could hardly avoid doing some household chores; if they could manage this, they were not seen as entitled to full compensation from their salaried jobs. The same reasoning affected one participant in the study; her right to full compensation was called into question after a heart attack when she was no longer able to work on the farm but was capable of performing some household tasks.

The Social Insurance Agency's exclusive focus on salaried work has thus created problems for women, since it does not account for unpaid work that is important for society as well as individuals and that cannot be circumvented. As previously mentioned, women today continue to have primary responsibility for home and children, even when they are ill (Statistics Sweden 2012b). They also assume greater responsibility for ill and aging family members. As is the case with regard to work-related injuries, Swedish physicians providing certification of illness should be aware that if they mention a woman's family and domestic

---

19 The mother of one of the authors of this book, married to a farmer, never forgot the humiliation she experienced when the small sick leave sum she received as a housewife was taken away because her husband was also eating the meal she had prepared when the inspector arrived. Despite lengthy, difficult periods of illness she never applied for sick leave again.

responsibilities she runs the risk of being denied compensation – a risk that hardly affects men.

Men's violence against women

The impact of the couple relationship on mental as well as physical health issues, stressed repeatedly above, was apparent for most women in our study. Several described husbands who set limits on their personal freedom in the work force and in social contacts. Some felt dominated in ways that impacted every aspect of their life. The husband's controlling behavior and their accommodation to it made them feel nervous, depressed, and fatigued. When they did not know what their husbands would do next, they lost control over everyday life, creating a growing dependence on his opinions and behavior. We define such a situation as emotional abuse, a term one woman herself used.[20] For some women, this situation continued into old age. As mentioned previously, however, a couple of them eventually managed, despite their husband's protests, to escape by divorcing or moving out. Because the balance of power in the marriage then changed – to the women's advantage – their health and quality of life improved rapidly.

A large survey of violence against women was conducted in Sweden in 1999. It demonstrated that even in this relatively egalitarian society, many women lack control at home, whether of resources or their own bodies. Of previously married or cohabiting women, 48 percent reported controlling behavior from their former partners, e.g. denying them financial responsibility and checking their contacts, while 12 percent reported such behavior from their present partners. For actual abuse the figures were 35 percent and 11 percent respectively (Lundgren et al. 2002). The numbers show that some of the oppressed women had succeeded in extracting themselves from these destructive situations.

Until 1982 only the woman herself, not an outsider, could press charges for violence in a couple's relationship (Dahlberg et al. 1990). Rape within marriage was not criminalized in Sweden until 1965, and only in the 1980s did rape come to be regarded as a serious, violent crime. Not until the 1990s did men's violence against women, including emotional, physical, and sexual abuse, draw attention as a

---

20 We actively sought to include a woman who had been physically abused in this study, but none of those we asked was willing or had the energy to participate.

social problem and a public health issue. At this time society assumed greater responsibility for assisting abused women and the term "men's violence against women" came into general use, rather than labels like "family dispute" or "domestic disturbance".[21]

The so-called Women's Protection reform (1998) made it possible for women to seek a restraining order against men who abused them. The protection offered to female victims of violence, whether within the home or outside it, nevertheless remains inadequate in present-day Sweden. Every year women are murdered by their partners or former partners, some after being denied safeguards in the form of a restraining order or protected identity.

One factor making it difficult to draw attention to domestic violence against women is the clear distinction between public and private spheres that has been, and continues to be, the norm in Swedish society. This attitude makes it possible to hide whatever goes on behind closed doors, resulting in silence about beatings and other forms of abuse, even when the woman seeks medical attention. Shame and guilt feelings, apprehension about encountering prejudice from the physician and other authorities, and fear that the violence will escalate if anything comes out are some reasons women keep quiet (Hamberg et al. 1998). Similarly, victims of rape and other kinds of sexual abuse outside the family have often refrained from revealing what has occurred or filing a police report. A sense of vulnerability within the justice system is a contributing factor in both situations. Even when charges are filed, many cases are closed without completing a proper investigation and four out of five do not come to trial (Lindgren 2013). If they do, the burden of proof often rests on the woman, who may herself be blamed for what occurred. Mitigating circumstances for the abusive man could be that the woman had behaved in a manner he found provocative. In rape cases outside the home, a woman's conduct and attire, or the perception that her refusal was not sufficiently clear, can still be held against her and viewed as a contributing factor to the crime.

Sexualized violence and healthcare

Medical science remained uninterested in men's violence against women for a long time. During the 1960s, for instance, the National

---

21 These terms nevertheless continue to appear, for instance in police reports, disguising the fact that the usual scenario is men beating their wives, live-in lovers, former wives or lovers, or mothers, and that violence cuts across the social spectrum.

Board of Health and Welfare opposed the criminalization of rape within marriage with the argument that women might take advantage of the law during divorce proceedings (Brunnberg 1985).[22] Thus the country's chief agency for public health prioritized the private and legal interests of men rather than the health of women. In reports on public health that were published regularly, men's violence against women was often excluded from the statistics.[23]

Medicine has thus been reluctant to acknowledge that this type of violence is a vitally important issue for women's health; awareness, strategies for treatment, and assistance to victims are still lacking in the healthcare system. The women's shelter movement, staffed by volunteers and feminist researchers, have instead drawn attention to the phenomenon and established the extent and significance of the violence (Eliasson 1997; Lundgren et al. 2002; ROKS 2011; 2012). Their work has counteracted common stereotypes, such as that most perpetrators are immigrants, have alcohol problems or are poorly educated. Research has also identified the process by which violence is "normalized" so that women remain in abusive relationships: increasing isolation in which threats and beatings eventually seem routine and the woman begins to believe she has brought them on herself. By alternating between violence and kindness, the man binds the woman to him more and more tightly (Lundgren 1993). One woman in our study gave a revealing account of this oscillation between emotional abuse and the release of tension (see Chapter 2).

Emotional and physical abuse and other forms of sexualized violence[24] are known to lie behind many different illnesses that affect women as well as leading to long-term sick leaves (Helweg-Larsen and Kruse 2003; Wijma et al. 2007; Thomsson 2013). Their self-esteem vanishes and they find themselves in a state of chronic tension leading to fatigue, pain, stomach upset, and depression (Lundgren 2002; Wijma et al. 2007; Socialstyrelsen 2014). To regain their health they need help finding words to describe their experiences and thereby gain a

---

22   When we attempted to track down the document, the National Board of Health and Welfare informed us that this particular item had disappeared.
23   When these figures were included, at the urging of women doctors and researchers, they were under-reported and disguised the fact that men's violence against women is often recurring, while occasional violence in public places between unacquainted men was presented as a far greater problem.
24   The umbrella term "sexualized violence" incorporates male-female battery, rape and other forms of sexual violence, including against children, and sexual harassment. Prostitution and violent pornography are usually included under this rubric. Prostitution is not, however, illegal in Sweden, although the purchase of sexual services is.

better understanding of what they have gone through; they need to rebuild self-esteem and the belief that they have a right to a life of their own. These goals, along with providing physical protection from violence, comprise the core mission of the Swedish women's shelter movement.[25] In healthcare it is necessary to identify and provide assistance to these women and be aware that violence also occurs in lesbian relationships.

In recent years there has been increased awareness of the large number of victims of trafficking in Sweden. Women are lured to Sweden, especially from Eastern Europe, the Baltic states, and Asia, with the promise of work, but end up being forced into prostitution. To date Swedish law provides very little protection to these victimized women, whose situation is extremely precarious.

Summary

Feminist criticism of medical science has often focused on the fact that men – and usually white, middle-class, heterosexual men at that – have been and continue to be seen as the norm.[26] Many examples provided in this chapter demonstrate that medical research and practice are not "neutral and genderless" (Risberg 2004). Consequently women's health issues have often been neglected. When seeking medical attention several women in this study discovered that physicians frequently lacked knowledge of their real-life situation and the workload they had to manage, nor did they ask questions that might have given the women an opportunity to explain. As a result their symptoms and ailments were not recognized and adequately treated. Some of them did, however, encounter consideration and a sympathetic ear from the doctor. This had helped them find the strength to accomplish what they felt needed to be done and occasionally provided an opportunity for the rest they needed.

There is reason to believe that ignorance of women's everyday lives remains great in the medical profession (Hölge-Hazelton and Malterud 2009). In Sweden, this applies particularly to migrants, women of color,

---

25 Women's shelters are currently located in cities and towns throughout Sweden. The National Centre for Knowledge on Men's Violence Against Women at Uppsala University offers assistance through a hot line and serves as a research and teaching center focusing on violence against women and ways to combat it.

26 At the same time, feminist research has often drawn on the situation of heterosexual middle-class Caucasian women in the western world, ignoring the experiences of all other women.

those living in poverty, and women in late middle age, a time when many suffer physical and/or emotional strain or are injured on the job while also having to cope with caregiving responsibilities in private life. When explanations for their illnesses are sought in reproductive biology or psychological state of mind, there is a major risk that important circumstances in life and at work, as well as actual illnesses, will be overlooked. Such ignorance disempowers women with regard to their own health.

Knowledge of the ways in which power issues, norms, and values affect health needs to be integrated into medical science and healthcare. A growing body of medical research demonstrates the direct impact of life circumstances on biology and the strong connection between health and equality in society (Pickett and Wilkinson 2009; Getz et al. 2011; McEwan and Getz 2013).

13

Everyday Life and Health

When the women described their daily lives, happiness and fortitude as well as suffering and struggle were in evidence, in varying proportions from person to person and in different phases of individual lives. In this chapter, we return to experiences that have been mentioned in earlier chapters, placing them in a broader context. We begin with symptoms common to many of the women. Although they are familiar, the healthcare system has paid little attention to them and they have often been seen as a sign of "the way women are," as essentialist characteristics. We also discuss what we term "strategies for maintaining health".

Common symptoms

Fatigue

Almost all the women described periods of fatigue that they ascribed to excessive work demands, too much responsibility, and a sense of never being able to do enough. This applied to both unpaid and paid work. In the private sphere, having total responsibility for the household and around-the-clock caregiving duties was experienced as especially exhausting. Women with dominating husbands felt a special kind of fatigue.

Even if it was prolonged, however, fatigue was not seen as an illness, but rather as a normal condition and nothing to complain about. The women were so used to being tired that they sometimes misinterpreted symptoms of serious illness and delayed seeking medical attention. For some, constant exhaustion had led to profound anxiety and a sense of powerlessness.

Fatigue remains common among young and middle-aged women. In an article drawing on interviews with young women, a British researcher summarized her results with the telling title, "My health is all right, I'm just tired all the time" (Popay 1992: 99). These women considered the demands of family life to be the primary reason for their fatigue, and like the women in our study, they saw it as something they simply had to put up with. It was also difficult for them to make their partners understand their need for rest. The researcher concluded: "If chronic and severe tiredness is a persistent feature of fulfilling the mother and wife role then it is to be expected that women will feel under pressure to cope with this too, and not to complain" (Popay 1992: 117).

Our study describes a correlation between satisfaction in the marital relationship and the woman's degree of fatigue. We also observed that fatigue in elderly women can by no means always be ascribed solely to age or illness. Just as with younger women, it is often a sign that they have taken on, or been burdened with, more than their strength can bear. In recent years in Sweden, cutbacks at care facilities for the elderly have reduced the number of places available, resulting in increased demands on family members, almost always women. We consider it completely unreasonable to expect an older person to be on call around the clock in the home.

Compulsive sensitivity

Whether in the public or private sphere, much of the women's work involved paying attention to the wellbeing of those around them. After many years of "practice," sensitivity to the needs and feelings of others could become an internal compulsion some women were unable to resist, making them increasingly likely to put others' needs before their own. We call this state of mind "compulsive sensitivity". It could evolve in a variety of situations and relationships, not least among women working in healthcare. Being attuned at all times to the needs of others was an emotional strain but also led to physically demanding work and the inability to rest or relax. Exhaustion, and when caregiving took place in the home, isolation, made the women gradually lose track of what was reasonable or "normal." If they tried to set limits on their efforts they were overcome by guilt feelings, as described so well by the woman who for years could not bring herself to insist that her bedridden and demanding husband be moved to a care facility. Outside intervention might have facilitated this.

The women viewed compulsive sensitivity as their own fault – that was simply the way they were. This perception appears to have been shared by those around them, so the women themselves were held accountable for not being able to stop "sacrificing themselves." By contrast, we see compulsive sensitivity as a consequence of overwhelming, unshared caregiving responsibilities, with little control over the workload and conditions and scant acknowledgment from others. Gendered expectations and norms were an underlying cause; financial constraints might worsen the situation, making it difficult to arrange for relief.

Emotional and physical exhaustion, sleep disorders, and pain in muscles and joints were outcomes the women themselves described. Research on work conditions has established that, compared to others, individuals under great emotional pressure on the job have an elevated pain threshold (Theorell et al. 1993). When doing physical labor, they presumably pay less attention to the body's warning signs, leading to an increased risk of developing chronic illness. Psychological symptoms brought on by a heavy workload may be ignored for a long time and eventually cause chronic fatigue or depression. We think it likely that compulsive sensitivity was a contributing factor in the cardiovascular diseases that struck several of the women in our study (compare Lennartsson et al. 2013). Women working at stressful healthcare jobs have a higher than average risk of developing and dying from cardiovascular disease (Järvholm and Reutervall 2012).

As general practitioners, we have encountered many women, young as well as old, who describe similar feelings of inner compulsion and are exhausted by the enormous burden of caring for others that is the outcome. Like the women in the study, they blame themselves, their attitude, their "womanliness." The healthcare system has often seen these women as choosing to play the role of martyr. The current notion that people are responsible for their own health may contribute to this perception. Recognizing compulsive sensitivity and gendered expectations as its cause provides a better understanding of these women and their situation and thus a greater likelihood that the healthcare system can intervene.[27]

Guilt

Guilt feelings were mentioned repeatedly in the women's accounts. They examined and reprimanded themselves for mistakes they had made

---

27 For a more detailed description of compulsive sensitivity as revealed in the women's accounts and ways this concept may be applied in the healthcare system, see Forssén, Carlstedt and Mörtberg 2005.

or things they had failed to do in relation to others and themselves. Those around them had also passed judgment and assigned guilt, and the prevailing wisdom of experts might lead to self-accusations.

The women were particularly hard on themselves when it came to their children. Healthcare workers had sometimes contributed to or brought on guilt feelings by blaming them for a difficult labor and delivery, the death of a child, or "inappropriate" feelings while breastfeeding. When the children were small, many women felt inadequate, a perception that remained painful to contemplate. Suffering brought on by guilt feelings was often private and not shared by their husbands. Quite the contrary: the women might feel guilty about problems between the children and their father because they considered themselves to have failed, or were accused of failing at the task of creating family harmony.

In her research on young, well-educated women in Sweden during the 1990s, the psychologist Ylva Elvin-Nowak encountered guilt feelings that are virtually identical in scope and content to those expressed by the women in our study. Elvin-Nowak refers to "everyday guilt" and to guilt as a way of living when women do not have the time and energy for their children that they feel they should. At the same time guilt is perceived as self-evident, something all mothers must live with (Elvin-Nowak 1999: 49). Neither then nor now have fathers been held accountable in the same way mothers are for how the children are doing.

Several women in our study blamed themselves for the unequal division of labor with regard to housework and childcare – they had not fought hard enough to correct the imbalance. If they had tried to bring about change they might attribute their husbands' lack of responsiveness to their own difficulty letting go of responsibility (compare Magnusson 1997; 2008). "My own fault" was a feeling that came up again and again.

The women's experiences demonstrate the importance of social norms for how guilt feelings arise; when perceptions of right and wrong changed, the burden of guilt could sometimes be lifted. This was the case, for instance, concerning childcare and childrearing when a rigid model governed by rules eventually was replaced by a more open and permissive way of seeing things. Other changes could make guilt feelings even worse. The divorced mother who kept the children away from their indifferent father – the right decision according to the standards of the period – later found that opinion had shifted: all children were now believed to need contact with both parents. Similarly, the woman married to the principal of a school who had followed the convention of the time and been a stay-at-home wife, had asked herself in recent years whether she should feel guilty about this now that all women were expected to have salaried employment. The norm that women should remain composed and not "make a fuss" that came out in interviews has also changed to some degree. Nowadays people are expected to assert themselves and claim their rights, although women are still held responsible for maintaining domestic harmony (Magnusson 1997; 2008). Thus it seems that no matter what women do, it may be considered wrong. Overall, it is apparent that for many women, guilt has been, and is, a control mechanism that hampers them from paying attention to their own needs.

Worry

Worry was a major drain on the women. They worried about unwanted pregnancies, children, born and unborn, other family members, difficulties with their spouses, money problems, becoming ill or not having enough energy, difficulties at the workplace and harassment. Those who had lived through war described anxiety and apprehension that never completely let up.

Like feelings of guilt, worry about children was usually private; it arose during close daily contact that no one else shared. Sometimes the women worried about the atmosphere in the home or father-child relationships where they felt caught in the middle without being able to influence the situation. They worried about their husbands' illnesses, which required them to assume the work of caregiving and rehabilitation. They might also worry about their spouses' behavior, as in the case of the woman who was afraid her husband would set the house on fire by smoking in bed. The term "care-as-worry" was coined to suggest the indissoluble connection between caring for family members, especially children, and worry about them (van Manen 2002: 262). Although this researcher does not consider gender issues, we view this in that context given that caregiving around the world is primarily done by women. This term may also be applied to salaried work, for instance in healthcare, where women hold most of the jobs.

As described by study participants, worry and the reasons for it counteract the perception that women are constitutionally anxious and nervous. Worry was neither a personal characteristic nor associated with innate "womanliness." It did, however, reflect women's great responsibility for the wellbeing of others and in some cases economic privation and the risk of physical violence. In Sweden today 50 percent of single mothers, a group that is often financially strapped and at risk for violence from ex-partners, describe themselves as worried much of the time (Statistics Sweden 2012b).

Shame

A deep-seated feeling that many women experienced was that they did not "measure up." This lack of self-esteem was not tied to social class or success in life, though some women mentioned that growing up in poverty and having little education could intensify the sensation.

Closely related to the sense of not measuring up was shame. Most women recalled realizing in their youth that their bodies were considered shameful. Menstruation was a taboo subject, viewed as nasty, not to mention sexual activity. The woman who became pregnant out of wedlock still dreamed about the disgrace fifty years later. Shame had made her, like the woman who had a baby after a divorce, deal with the experience in silence.

The women who had been subjected to sexual harassment also felt shame. One of them saw the harassment as proof of her low status as a cleaner. The memory of humiliation remained at the time of the interviews, though it had become less intense once a shift in social attitudes made it possible to talk about such matters. Over time, women gradually realized they were not alone in their experiences.

Women whose marriages were unhappy felt ashamed that they had not managed to establish a good relationship. Shame prevented them from talking to others about this and made it more difficult for them to move out or get a divorce. They also kept silent for fear that no one would understand, which would confirm their sense of inferiority. Telling someone would also bring their humiliation into the open, perhaps to people not intended to know, and as a result not even friends ever found out. Such feelings have continued to prevent many women from sharing their stories. Shame-induced silence was also the response to traumatic experiences or a sense of failure in connection with childbearing.

Although attitudes are now more open about women's bodies and sexuality, even young women may nevertheless have negative feelings about their sexual organs. Having one's period is still seen as embarrassing; it must be hidden and leave no trace.[28] A report from a Swedish clinic for young people describes young women as often conveying "the sense that their sexual organs were unclean," as lacking

---

28 This message is prominent in advertisements for sanitary pads and tampons but can also be traced back several thousand years. Passages in the Bible give a detailed description of the impurity of menstrual blood; physical contact with a menstruating woman also makes others unclean. See Leviticus Ch. 15, v. 19-24.

words for their external genitalia and having insufficient knowledge of their bodies and their sexuality (Hovelius 1996: 112). The increasing number of cosmetic operations to breasts and genitalia also suggests that women do not think they measure up as they are.

Loneliness

The women described loneliness in contrasting ways. It could stem from being responsible for group consensus and constantly responding to others' needs while one's own needs were ignored, a type of loneliness primarily found within marriage, or from not feeling needed by anyone, which most often applied in the absence of close relatives.

Many women found it painful that they could not talk to and share their thoughts with their husbands. They felt abandoned during pregnancy and after miscarriages, in their daily and nightly dealings with children, and because they bore sole responsibility for making everything run smoothly. Years spent at home with young children could lead to isolation. Women might also be isolated if their husbands set limits on social contact.

The convention in social life and community activities of doing things as a couple contributed to some women's isolation, whether married or not; unmarried women sometimes felt they were disregarded. When children, grandchildren, and husbands were the dominant topic of conversation among female friends, some were left out. Not having the resources or energy to entertain in the expected manner also meant that some women became cut off from friends. In the work force, women in supervisory positions sometimes encountered disrespect from men and women who reported to them and might have no peer group for support.

Overall, the women's stories underscore that external circumstances do not always reveal or account for feelings of loneliness and isolation.

Strategies for health

In the following section we highlight some strategies for maintaining health or strategies of resistance that came out in the women's accounts. They demonstrate that the women were aware of what was necessary for them to feel good and stay healthy.

A room of one's own

The first strategy, which has been mentioned previously, we call "a room of one's own," an expression borrowed from Virginia Woolf's 1929 essay of the same title. Woolf emphasizes that women are entitled to autonomy and discusses the right to, and options for, work and creativity separate from the family (Woolf 1929). In the following, we relate this concept to health.

For two of the women who never married, this was a conscious choice that enabled them to live and work with the freedom they desired, a freedom that was necessary for their wellbeing. Several married women who were at the hub of family life also described trying to find a private place for rest and attending to their own needs. The right to such a place was never self-evident, however, and might require challenging a spouse as well as the conventions of the day. The possibility of a physical space of one's own was also dependent on the size of the residence, where the children's needs often came first. For two of the women, a separate room was necessary to protect them from the domineering control, both physical and emotional, of their husbands.

Other ways of establishing a kind of separation while surrounded by others included doing handiwork, taking a break to smoke, and writing letters or diary entries. Louise Waldén, who specializes in the history of technology, has pointed out that by embroidering, women create a free zone in an existence dominated by others' needs (Waldén 2005: 14). Smoking that serves this function has been described by sociologist Ann Oakley as a "smoke ring that shuts out others for a short while" (Oakley 1993: 136). This separation can – in the short run – give women whose daily lives are hard-pressed the energy to go on and thus be a way of taking responsibility for others, despite the well-known risks (Graham 1994: 102-123). In Sweden today, smoking is most common among low-income women, especially single mothers (Socialstyrelsen 2012).

For many women, salaried work was an important "room of one's own" that gave them the right, and the obligation, to leave home. Going to and from work provided an opportunity to let thoughts roam freely, as could the occasional hour alone on the job, even if the work itself was not always stimulating. The women also had close ties to fellow workers. Meeting friends, being involved with clubs and organizations, or attending cultural events were other ways to escape the demands of always being available to others and were sometimes easier to implement than uninterrupted time at home.

Thus the women's need for a room of their own was not solely about a physical space; it concerned time to oneself and an autonomous life separate from home and family. This longing did not disappear when the children moved out. In old age women also needed to create this kind of separation, in particular those who cared for ailing husbands or other relatives. This is still the case for many older women.

The issue of a room of one's own is still relevant for younger women as well. The guilt that mothers feel about not spending enough time with their children – although they usually devote more time to children than fathers do – makes it difficult for them to insist on their right to a private space. Furthermore, even when they are not physically present, they are expected to leave their cell phones switched on and be reachable at all times. These constraints, both internal and external, make it imperative that the healthcare system pay attention to women's need for seclusion and undisturbed time to themselves and support their efforts to create such havens. The social norm that couples always share a bedroom may also need to be re-evaluated without construing this as a threat to the relationship.[29]

Self-determination

Being able to make their own decisions was an issue that came up early for many of the women. Some had succeeded, in whole or in part, in setting their own course, for instance the artist who at age sixteen deliberately burned the pea soup to escape continued running of the household, an act that had great significance for her life and happiness. Others were unable to escape assuming responsibility for the household and the family while still young. Limited economic resources could also be a barrier to getting an education or pursuing other goals.

The artist and a few others retained control of their daily lives by remaining single. Others felt that marriage had brought them more decision-making power because their financial circumstances improved and they could have a home of their own. Most women wanted to continue working outside the home after marriage, not least to retain a degree of financial independence. For two with strenuous, low-paying jobs, however, staying home seemed to offer more control over time and work tasks, even if it meant being financially dependent on their husbands. A prerequisite for feeling good about themselves was nevertheless that their husbands treated them with respect and

---

29 For a more detailed discussion of "a room of one's own" as a strategy for health, see Forssén and Carlstedt 2006.

they could determine how money was spent. In unequal relationships the woman's assertion of her own rights could instead lead to more controlling behavior on the part of the husband.

In the work force, self-determination was often limited, especially for those who worked in healthcare, in industrial kitchens, or industry. Those who could make independent decisions about their work hours and influence work conditions emphasized how important this was in boosting energy and promoting work satisfaction.

Decision-making power with regard to sexuality and reproduction was particularly significant for the women's health. Legislation and prevailing social attitudes restricted access to contraceptives; the possibility of control over childbearing also depended on the dynamics of the marital relationship. Since that time, Swedish women have successively achieved greater autonomy with regard to sexuality and childbearing. Recently, however, certain groups have begun calling into question the right to abortion, guaranteed by law since 1975. Banning abortion is a threat to women's health, as the example of Romania establishes: when such a ban was implemented, maternal mortality rates, linked with childbirth, doubled, and more than quadrupled following an illegal abortion despite the birth rate remaining the same (WHO 1992).

Attaining self-determination was thus both an achievement and a balancing act. The desire for control over one's own life could cause conflict with others and might have to be adjusted to accommodate caregiving responsibilities. Recognizing these complexities is essential in efforts to help women become more autonomous.[30]

Making a contribution

The women described wanting and needing to work; it brought them satisfaction and pleasure, whether or not it was for pay. "Having the energy to work" was often synonymous with being healthy and feeling good. That they had no choice but to keep working could also make them stronger, since it was a sign of their important, even indispensable role. Giving meaning to everyday life and creating a pleasant environment for others and themselves was the goal and significance of much work. This was illustrated by women who were proud of what they had accomplished by taking care of the children

---

30 This is the background to the title of our joint dissertation based on the interviews, *Between Responsibility and Power* (Carlstedt and Forssén 1999).

and giving them a good home. Another recalled that her competence as an engineer created job opportunities for others.[31]

Being busy all the time with meaningful work – at home, in the work force, or both – could thus provide a sense of wellbeing and keep the women healthy. They used expressions like "Life is best when you're hard at work." By way of comparison, research on workforce conditions has established through the demand-control model that high and meaningful demands accompanied by the knowledge of being capable and mastering the situation has a positive effect on health (Karasek and Theorell 1990).

Through work the women could also at times control, reduce, or forget about aches and pains. They mentioned not having time to consider how they were feeling or worry about themselves. In an article titled "Work as heaven from pain" the anthropologist Mary-Jo Good presents similar results in which clearly defined, goal-oriented tasks were found to soothe pain, and caring for others could divert attention from one's own suffering. Based on these findings she questions the conventional discourse that characterizes (salaried) work as primarily "a stressful source of pain." Instead she emphasizes that the effect on health depends on whether or not the work is perceived as meaningful (Good 1992).

Despite a heavy workload both inside and outside the home, a number of women had also devoted themselves to volunteer work. They wanted to make a contribution beyond the private sphere by becoming involved in the peace movement, establishing a women's shelter, fighting poverty at home and abroad, or working for a political party. This involvement was significant for their self-respect even if it was not always fully appreciated by those around them.

Culture and creative work

The artist in our study had felt a deep inner drive to create; this was as necessary to her as the air she breathed. When she continued painting in old age despite progressively deteriorating eyesight she called these works her "survival pictures." But there were other women as well who wanted to express their personalities, their creativity, and their capabilities in ways that could be seen or heard. Playing an instrument, singing, or dancing was essential to some. Several kept diaries or wrote letters, which provided them with time for reflection.

---

31 For a more detailed description of these strategies linked to mothering and paid employment, see Forssén and Carlstedt 2007, 2008.

One woman referred to "getting it down in writing," for herself and for later generations.

Beauty and sensory pleasure were important in daily life. Caring for flowers, ironing a cloth, or mangling the linens could provide moments of gratification through an awareness of color, fragrance, or a smooth surface. By doing handiwork the women made their homes more attractive and welcoming. The creative process itself forced them to focus on beauty in a concentrated way; the product provided comfort and pleasure in a life dominated by duties. We believe these efforts to bring beauty to everyday life contributed to the wellbeing of the entire family, but we are not aware of any research that connects this type of work, usually done by women, to health issues. Today, when many Swedish homes have become status symbols to be shown off, it may be more difficult to be satisfied by a kind of beauty that costs little and stems from individual creativity.

Regardless of their background, the women found it important to participate in local cultural activities. They attended the theater, concerts, and art exhibits and participated in book clubs. These experiences strengthened and comforted them, bolstered their self-confidence when they recognized themselves in what was depicted, and placated feelings of loneliness. A personal religious faith offered some women reconciliation and comfort. A sense of fellowship within the congregation was also meaningful.

Some women expressed a strong need to laugh and tease in order to get through daily life. Humor counteracted loneliness and physical pain, made it easier to deal with strenuous work, and helped them relax and rest. Banter and joking came up at work or with relatives and good friends.

That the women, regardless of social class or level of education, attributed such significance to beauty, cultural activities, and humor came as a surprise to us. Their reactions demonstrated that the connection between these factors and health has been undervalued.[32]

As we see it, medical research and treatment should be directed more toward strengthening the inner resources for maintaining health that are unique to each individual, drawing on that person's awareness and preferences, rather than unilaterally focusing on the risk of illness.

---

[32] For a more detailed description of humor, beauty and culture as personal health resources, see Forssén 2007.

Conclusion

One starting point of our research was the realization that the word "work" is often associated only with salaried employment and that much of what women have done, and continue to do, thus remains unseen. For that reason, drawing attention to women's unpaid work by describing what it encompassed, its conditions and its significance became an important goal. Most of the women in our study had devoted a considerable part of their lives to unpaid work, some with daily household and caring responsibilities for as many as 70 years. In addition, the majority had been employed for long periods, some for nearly half a century. Many had also devoted a number of years to the work of bearing children. Both the scope and duration of the women's work activities exceeded what is usually encompassed by the concepts of "working age" or "active working life", which ordinarily include neither providing care in their domestic lives nor work undertaken after the usual age of retirement.

During the lives of the study's participants, Sweden underwent a profound transformation from one of Europe's most impoverished nations, ruled by the privileged few, to a democratically governed welfare state where class differences successively diminished. The society the women grew up and lived in was nevertheless segregated according to gender; men had more power than women, and women encountered far more economic and legal restrictions than men did. These factors, combined with the prevailing view of women's innate nature and capabilities, determined the type of work they were expected to do. All women had to take these matters into account, regardless of whether they personally concurred with prevailing norms and standards.

As women achieved more rights and as perceptions about their place in society became less rigid – to a large degree through their own efforts – the power relationship between women and men shifted in women's favor. One of the most significant changes was access to contraceptives and safe abortions, giving women greater control of their sexuality and their childbearing. Another was the expectation that all women, regardless of marital status or social class, would find salaried employment and support themselves, which replaced the ideal of the housewife supported by her husband. Beginning in the 1970s, political reforms, including parental leave with pay and the right to subventioned daycare for all children, facilitated this social reconfiguration. The outcome has been a more equal distribution of work between women and men; both women's participation in the labor market and men's participation in housework and caregiving have increased since the reforms went into effect.

Even so, as we have stressed repeatedly in this book, the goal of equal opportunities for women and men has not been reached. Men continue to have more power than women, whether politically, economically, or in the labor market; expectations and demands placed on women and men remain different. Only recently has the extent and significance of men's violence against women drawn attention. Class differences are once again on the rise and certain groups are marginalized or looked down upon based on ethnicity, religion, skin color or gender identity. On the lowest rung of the ladder, and often exploited, are migrants and refugees.

Although the primary focus of our study was on the work history of participants and its relation to health issues, we also gained insight into other important aspects of their lives. We were surprised by the strength, joy, and vitality they conveyed despite circumstances and experiences that often were trying, even grim. Most of them had solved problems and managed and overcome heavy workloads and other difficulties without losing heart. As they looked back on their lives at the time of the interviews, they were content and often proud of what they had accomplished. They also made a conscious effort to come to terms with matters that still caused pain. For some, knowing they had given their children a good home was particularly important; for others, it was the conviction that they had performed well on the job. In addition, many of the women felt life was good to them in old age and were hopeful about the future. Still, for some, sorrow and disappointment did not let up, making it difficult to retroactively focus on the positive or look forward with confidence.

The skills and training in housework, caregiving, and relational work that most women had acquired and practiced in their lives were not only important in that generation, but will continue to be needed in the future because they respond to people's fundamental needs: food, personal hygiene, making ends meet, and taking care of each other. We call these "survival skills", which especially in various crisis situations, such as economic privation, natural catastrophe or war, can be of major, sometimes vital significance. As we have noted previously, women's skills in these areas should not be regarded as a female "virtue" or an inborn characteristic, but rather be valued and respected as acquired competence. Passing on these skills to both women and men is fundamental to establishing gender equality and for maintaining health.

Many of the women had learned, over the years, what was important for health and wellbeing, their own and others', and recounted ways in which they had kept their strength up and found pleasure in daily life. Health was not only a medical matter but concerned life in its entirety. Some women described feeling healthy despite chronic illness; in general, the perception of good health was often connected to work, paid and unpaid, assuming the work was meaningful and they could influence its content and scope. Other significant factors included self-determination with regard to important choices in life, access to "a room of one's own," money of one's own, encountering respect for work performed, creating and experiencing culture and beauty, and receiving care, love, and friendship from others. As women, they had sometimes been forced to struggle hard to fulfill such needs. A fundamental insight that participants in our study conveyed is that power over one's own body, one's work situation and one's responsibilities is essential for women's prospects of conquering illness and maintaining health.

APPENDIX

Significant Dates in Women's History in Sweden

1842	Obligatory six-year primary school for both girls and boys
1845	Equal rights of inheritance for women and men
1846	Unmarried women (including widows and divorcées) allowed to work in handicrafts and trades
1858	Unmarried women attain majority at age 25 by registering at court of law
1859	Women may work as primary school teachers and in lower-level positions in the public sector
1864	Unmarried women are granted the same legal rights to conduct business as men
1864	Wife-beating is outlawed
1870	Women may take matriculation examinations after private study
1872	Women gain the right to choose whom they will marry
1873	Women are admitted to universities with the right to take an academic degree, though not in theology or law
1884	Establishment of the Fredrika Bremer Society, Sweden's first feminist organization, named for the well-known author and champion of women's rights
1884	Unmarried women attain majority at age 21
1886	Establishment of the first women's occupational organization, the Swedish Midwives Association
1886	First women's trade union, the Seamstress Union in Lund
1888	Establishment of the Women's Workers' Association, the first organization in the socialist women's movement
1888	The first woman physician, Karolina Widerström, receives her medical degree
1900	Prohibition against women working underground in quarries or mines
1901	Right to four weeks unpaid leave at the birth of a child

1902	Establishment of the Women's Trade Union, comprised primarily of seamstresses
1902	First organization promoting women's suffrage, with members from several political parties
1904	The Women's Trade Union is incorporated in LO (Landsorganisationen), the umbrella organization for all Swedish trade unions
1905	Children born out of wedlock inherit from their mothers on an equal basis with children born within marriage
1909	Universal suffrage for men at age 24
1909	Prohibition against women working at night in industry
1909	Introduction of public intermediate (post-primary) schools open to both sexes and qualifying graduates for secondary school
1910	Women gain the right to work throughout the public sector
1910	Prohibition against disseminating information about or selling contraceptives
1914	Selma Lagerlöf becomes the first female member of the Swedish Academy (the body that awards the Nobel Prize in literature)
1915	Women may initiate divorce proceedings
1917	Law requiring that paternity of children born out of wedlock be established and that fathers pay child support
1918	Repeal of law requiring prostitutes to register with the police
1918	Women may be instructors or principals in public secondary schools
1921	First election in which women may vote
1921	Married women attain majority at age 21
1922	The first five women members of parliament take office
1923	Qualifications Law (Behörighetslagen) gives women and men equal access to jobs in the public sector except those involving physical violence (the military and the police)
1927	Public secondary schools are open to girls on an equal basis with boys
1931	Maternity insurance becomes available through certain private insurance companies, providing 20-42 days of paid sick leave in connection with childbirth and covering the midwife's fee
1935	Women and men receive the same retirement pensions
1936	Women working in the public sector receive the right to paid leave during pregnancy and after the birth of a child
1937	Equal pay for female and male primary school teachers

1938	Ban on contraceptive use and sale is lifted
1938	Need-based payment to new mothers to cover costs associated with giving birth
1938	Abortion is permitted under certain strictly regulated medical circumstances
1939	Engagement, marriage, pregnancy, and childbirth are no longer valid reasons for dismissal from jobs in the public sector
1944	Homosexuality is decriminalized
1946	Women and men have the right to equal pay in all public sector jobs except ecclesiastical and military positions
1947	First female cabinet minister
1948	Child supplement support is introduced
1949	Mothers, whether married or not, receive the right to become guardians of their children
1949	The phrase in the 1809 constitution referring to "native-born Swedish men" is changed to "Swedish citizens"
1951	Women may retain Swedish citizenship upon marriage to a foreign national
1955	Health insurance is nationalized; 90 days of income-based maternity leave
1955	Payment to new mothers is no longer need-based
1958	Women may be ordained in the Swedish Lutheran Church, although bishops are not obliged to perform the ceremony
1960	Women and men to receive equal pay for equal work
1962	Parliament supports the United Nations proclamation on equal pay for equal work
1964	The birth control pill becomes available in Sweden
1965	Rape within marriage is outlawed
1966	The IUD is permitted as a contraceptive device
1969	Equal rights are included in the national curriculum for primary school
1970	Establishment of first youth clinic for sex education
1970	Children born out of wedlock inherit from their fathers
1971	Joint taxation for married couples is eliminated
1974	Parental leave replaces maternity leave, giving parents the right to share paid (income-based) leave time (initially 6 months, thereafter incremental increases to 15 months in 2014); a base sum to mothers without an income
1975	New abortion law gives women sole decision-making rights and unrestricted access to abortion up to the 18th week of pregnancy

Appendix 171

1975	United Nations sponsors International Women's Year
1978	Sweden's first women's shelters open in Stockholm and Göteborg
1978	Corporal punishment of children is outlawed
1979	Parents of children under age 8 may reduce their work schedule to 6 hours a day
1979	Parliament passes a law guaranteeing workplace equality
1979	Homosexuality is no longer classified as an illness
1980	Female right of succession to the Swedish throne is reinstated after a hiatus of nearly 350 years
1980	Sexual discrimination in the workplace is outlawed
1980	JämO (Jämställdhetsombudsmannen), the Equality Ombudsman, is introduced; renamed DO (Diskriminerings-ombudsmannen), the Discrimination Ombudsman, in 2009
1982	Prohibition of pornographic performances in public places such as theaters and cinemas
1982	A third party may press charges in cases of domestic violence against women
1982	Increased legal safeguards for women and children in cases of incest and other sexual crimes
1984	Establishment of National Organisation for Women's Shelters
1987	Discrimination against homosexuals is outlawed
1988	Women may take out restraining orders on abusive men
1989	All work categories open to women, including the military
1991	New law on gender equality prohibits sexual harassment in the workplace
1994	Sweden's parliament becomes the most gender-balanced in the world, with 144 female members of a total of 349
1994	Introduction of registered partnerships for same-sex couples
1995	Introduction of the so-called "Daddy month" – the requirement that fathers take at least 30 days of parental leave
1995	Legal requirement that pay discrepancies between women and men be investigated at all work places
1998	Purchasing sexual services is outlawed
1998	Women's Protection Law introduced to combat men's violence against women
1998	Genital mutilation of women is prohibited
1999	HomO established (ombudsman to combat discrimination on the basis of sexual orientation)
1999	Possession of child pornography is prohibited
2003	Prohibition of hate speech directed against ethnic groups is expanded to include sexual orientation

2003	Gay couples who are registered partners may apply to become adoptive parents
2005	Lesbian couples who live together or are registered partners have the right to undergo artificial insemination
2006	Prohibition of discrimination or harassment of children and schoolchildren
2006	Establishment of National Centre for Knowledge on Men's Violence Against Women
2009	Same-sex marriage is legalized
2009	Discrimination against transgender identification or expression is outlawed
2009	The Social Welfare Agency no longer classifies transvestite, fetishist, or sadomasochistic behavior as illness
2010	Requirements for military service become gender-neutral
2011	Constitutional amendment to forbid discrimination on the basis of sexual orientation
2013	Repeal of law requiring sterilization of transsexuals

References

Allen, Isobel. (2005). Women doctors and their careers: what now? *British Medical Journal/BMJ*, 331, 569-572.
Arbetsskadekommissionen. (2012). *Förslag till en reformerad arbetsskadeförsäkring. En rapport från Arbetsskadekommissionen.* Rapport, 4 September.
Artazcoz, Lucia, Borrell, C., Benach, Joan, Cortès, I., and Rohlfs, I. (2004). Women, family demands and health: the importance of employment status and socioeconomic position. *Social Science & Medicine*, 59, 263-274.
Beck, Cheryl T. (2006). Pentadic cartography: Mapping birth trauma narratives. *Qualitative Health Research*, 16, 453-466.
——. (2011). A metaethnography of traumatic childbirth and its aftermath: Amplifying causal looping. *Qualitative Health Research*, 21, 301-311.
Beck, Cheryl T. and Watson, Sue. (2008). Impact of birth trauma on breast-feeding. A tale of two pathways. *Nursing Research*, 57, 228-236.
Beral, Valerie and Million Women Study Collaborators. (2003). Breast cancer and hormone-replacement therapy in the Million Women Study. *Lancet*, 362 (9382), 419-427.
Bewley, Susan and Cockburn, Jane. (2002). The unfacts of "request" caesarean section. *BJOG/ an International Journal of Obstetrics and Gynaecology*, 109 (6), 597-605.
Bjerén, Gunilla, Carlstedt, Gunilla, Elgqvist-Saltzman, Inga, Johansson, Annika, Liljeström, Rita and Sundström, Kajsa. (2009). *Livstider. Kvinnors liv under 1900-talet.* Stockholms universitet. Centrum för Genusstudiers skriftserie, 44.
Boalt, Carin. (1983). Tid för hemarbete. Hur lång tid då? In Brita Åkerman (ed.). *Den okända vardagen – om arbetet i hemmen.* Stockholm: Förlaget Akademilitteratur AB.
Bohlin, Rebecka. (2012). *De Osynliga. Om Europas fattiga arbetarklass.* Stockholm: Atlas Reportage.
Bohlin, Elsa. (1987). *Porträtt utan guldram.* Stockholm: Tidens Förlag.
Brunnberg, Eva. (1985). Ett möte mellan juridik och medicin. *Socialmedicinsk tidskrift*, 62, 380-387.
Bäckström, Taina and Wamala, Sarah. (2012). *Folkhälsan i Sverige. Årsrapport 2012.* Stockholm: The National Board of Health and Welfare/StatensFolkhälsoinstitut. http://www.folkhalsomyndigheten.

se/publicerat-material/publikationer/Folkhalsan-i-Sverige-Arsrapport-2012/
Callaghan, Glenn M., Chacon, C., Coles, C., Botts, J. and Laraway, Sean. (2008). An empirical evaluation of the diagnostic criteria for premenstrual dysphoric disorder. Problems with sex specificity and validity. *Women & Therapy*, 32, 1-21.
Carlstedt, Gunilla. (2009). "Man måste hela tiden arbeta" – en livsberättelse från 1900-talets Sverige. In Bjerén, Gunilla, Carlstedt, Gunilla, Elgqvist-Saltzman, Inga, Johansson, Annika, Liljeström, Rita. and Sundström, Kajsa. *Livstider. Kvinnoliv på 1900-talet*, pp. 21-68. Stockholms Universitet: Centrum för Genusstudiers skriftserie, 44.
Carlstedt, Gunilla and Forssén, Annika. (1999). *Mellan ansvar och makt. En diskussion om arbete, hälsa och ohälsa utifrån tjugo kvinnors livsberättelser.* [Dissertation with English summary.] Luleå: Luleå University of Technology, Department of Human Work Sciences.
Carlstedt, Gunilla and The Swedish Research Council's Committee for Gender Research. (2008). Gender in Medical Research Applications – A follow up study of the Swedish Research Council's awards in 2004. Stockholm: The Swedish Research Council. www.vr.se
Dahlberg, Anita, Nordborg, Gudrun and Wicklund, Elvy. (1990). *Kvinnors Rätt*. Stockholm: Tiden/Folksam.
Danielsson, Maria and Lindberg, Gudrun. (2001). Differences between men's and women's health: The old and new gender paradox. In Östlin, Piroska, Danielsson, Maria, Diderichsen, Finn, Härenstam, Annika and Lindberg, Gudrun. *Gender Inequalities in Health* (pp. 23-66). Boston: Harvard University Press.
Davies, Karen. (1987). Manlig tid och kvinnors verklighet. *Kvinnovetenskaplig tidskrift*, 8 (4), 26-38.
—. (1990). *Women, Time and the Weaving of the Strands of Everyday Life*. Aldershot: Avebury.
—. (2001). *Disturbing Gender: on the doctor-nurse relationship*. Lund: Lund Studies in Sociology.
Dick-Read, Grantly. (1933). *Natural Childbirth*. London: William Heinemann Medical Books.
Dresser, R. (1992). Wanted: Single, White Male for Medical Research. *Hastings Center Report*, 22, 24-29.
Eklund, Ulrika. (2010). *Jämställda sjukskrivningar – arbetsbok för kvalitetssäkrad sjukskrivningsprocess*. Stockholm: Sveriges kommuner och landsting/The Swedish Association of Local Authorities and Regions.
Elgqvist-Saltzman, Inga. (1994). Att vända på bilden. *Kvinnovetenskaplig tidskrift*, 15(4), 18-29.

References 175

Eliasson, Mona. (1997). *Mäns våld mot kvinnor. Misshandel. Våldtäkt. Dominans. Kontroll.* Stockholm: Natur och Kultur.
Elvin-Nowak, Ylva. (1999). *Accompanied by Guilt. Modern Motherhood the Swedish Way.* [Dissertation.] Stockholm: Stockholm University, Department of Psychology.
Elwér, Sofia. (2013). *Gender equality and health experiences: workplace patterns in Northern Sweden.* [Dissertation.] Umeå: Umeå University.
Eriksson, Nancy. (1964). *Bara en hemmafru. Ett debattinlägg om kvinnor i familjen.* Stockholm: Mauritzens bo0ktryckeri.
Fausto-Sterling, Anne. (2011). *Sex and Gender: Biology in a Social World.* London: Routledge.
Ferree, Myra M. (1976). Working-Class Jobs: Housework and Paid Work as Sources of Satisfaction. *Social Problems*, 23, 431-441.
Forssén, Annika. (2007). Humour, beauty and culture as personal health resources – experiences of elderly Swedish women. *Scandinavian Journal of Public Health*, 35, 228-234.
—. (2012). Lifelong Significance of Disempowering Experiences in Prenatal and Maternity Care: Interviews With Elderly Swedish Women. *Qualitative Health Research*, 22(11), 1536-1546.
Forssén, Annika and Carlstedt, Gunilla. (2001). Work, Health and Ill Health. New research makes women's experiences visible. *Scandinavian Journal of Primary Health Care*, 19, 154-157.
—. (2006). "It's heavenly to be alone!": A room of one's own as a health-promoting resource for women. Results from a qualitative study. *Scandinavian Journal of Public Health*, 34, 175-181.
—. (2007). Health-promoting aspects of a paid job: findings in a qualitative interview study with elderly women in Sweden. *Health Care for Women International*, 28, 909-929.
—. (2008). "You really do something useful with kids." Mothering and Experienced Health and Illness in a Group of Elderly Swedish Women. *Health Care for Women International*, 29, 1019-1039.
Forssén, Annika, Carlstedt, Gunilla and Mörtberg, Christina. (2005). Compulsive sensitivity – a consequence of caring: A qualitative investigation into women carers' difficulties in limiting their labors. *Health Care for Women International*, 26, 652-671.
Försäkringskassan. (2013). *Social Insurance in Figures.*
Gavanas, Anna. (2010). *Who Cleans the Welfare State? Migration, Informalization, Social Exclusion and Domestic Services in Stockholm.* Stockholm: Institutet för framtidsstudier.
Getz, Linn, Kirkengen, Anna-Louise and Ulvestad, Erling. (2011). The human biology – Saturated with experience. *Tidsskrift for Norsk Legeforening*, 131, 683-687.

Giorgi, Amadeo. (1985). Sketch of a psychological phenomenological method. In Amadeo Giorgi (ed.). *Phenomenology and Psychological Research* (pp. 8-22). Pittsburgh: Duquesne University Press.
Good, Mary-Jo D. (1992). Work as heaven from pain. In Mary-Jo Good, Brodwin Good and A. Kleinman (eds). *Pain as Human Experience: An Anthropological Perspective* (pp. 49-76). Berkeley and Los Angeles: University of California Press.
Graham, Hilary. (1994). Surviving by smoking. In Sue Wilkinson and Ceila Kitzinger (eds). *Women and Health: Feminist Perspectives* (pp. 102-123). London: Taylor & Francis.
Gustafsson, Rolf Å. and Szebehely, Marta. (2001). Women's health and changes in care for the elderly. In Östlin, Piroska, Danielsson, Maria, Diderichsen, Finn, Härenstam, Annika and Lindberg, Gudrun (eds). *Gender Inequalities in Health* (pp. 245-268). Boston: Harvard University Press.
Hamberg, Katarina. (2008). Gender bias in medicine. *Women's Health*, 4(3), 237-243.
Hamberg, Katarina, Johansson, Eva, Lindgren, Gerd and Westman, Göran. (1997). The impact of marital relationship on the rehabilitation process in a group of women with long-term musculoskeletal disorders. *Scandinavian Journal of Social Medicine*, 25, 17-25.
—. (1998). "I was always on guard" – An exploration of woman abuse in a group of women with musculoskeletal pain. *Family Practice*, 16(3), 238-244.
Hamberg, Katarina, Risberg, Gunilla, Johansson, Eva and Westman, Göran. (2002). Gender bias in physicians' management of neck pain: a study of the answers in a Swedish national examination. *Journal of Women's Health and Gender-based Medicine*, 11, 653-665.
Hamberg, Katarina, Risberg, Gunilla and Johansson, Eva E. (2004). Male and female physicians show different patterns of gender bias. A paper-case study of management of irritable bowel syndrome. *Scandinavian Journal of Public Health*, 32, 144-152.
Hammarström, Anne, Lehti, Arja, Danielsson, Ulla, Bengs, Carita and Johansson, Eva E. (2009). Gender-related explanatory models of depression: a critical evaluation of medical articles. *Public Health*, 123, 689-693.
Hammarström, Anne and Phillips, Susan. (2012). Gender inequity needs to be regarded as a social determinant of depressive symptoms: Results from the Northern Swedish cohort. *Scandinavian Journal of Public Health*, 40, 746-752.
Haraway, Donna. (1991). Situated knowledges: The science question in feminism and the privilege of partial perspective. In Donna Haraway (ed,). *Simians, Cyborgs, and Women: The Reinvention of Nature* (pp. 183-201). New York: Routledge.

References 177

Harryson, Lisa. (2013). *"An equal share, that's my medicine":   Work, gender relations and mental illness in a Swedish context.* [Dissertation.] Umeå: Umeå University.

Haug, Frigga. (1992). *Beyond Female Masochism: Memory-Work and Politics.* London and New York: Verso.

Helweg-Larsen, Karin and Kruse, Marie. (2003). Violence against women and consequent health problems: a register-based study. *Scandinavian Journal of Public Health*, 31, 51-57.

Hemström, Örjan. (2005). Health inequalities by wage income in Sweden: The role of work environment. *Social Science & Medicine*, 61, 637-647.

Hensing, Gunnel. (2012). Genusaspekter på socialförsäkringen – Om kvinnors och mäns sjukfrånvaro. In Försäkringskassan. *Kön, klass och etnicitet. Jämlikhetsfrågor i socialförsäkringen. Rapport från forskarseminariet i Umeå, 18-19 januari 2012.* Social Insurance Report 2012:4.

Hinze, Susan W. (2004). "Am I being oversensitive?" Women's experiences of sexual harassment during medical training. *Health*, 8, 101-127.

Hirdman, Yvonne. (1987). Konsten att vara kvinna. Stilleben, Sverige 1950. In Birgit Sawyer and Anita Göransson (eds). *Manliga strukturer och kvinnliga strategier. En bok till Gunhild Kyle* (pp. 292-307). Göteborg: Meddelanden från Historiska Institutionen, 33.

—. (1990). *The gender system: Theoretical reflections on the social subordination of women.* Study of Power and Democracy in Sweden. Uppsala: Maktutredningen.

Hirschbein, Laura D. (2006). Science, gender, and the emergence of depression in American psychiatry, 1952-1980. *Journal of the History of Medicine and Allied Sciences*, 61, 187-216.

Holm, Ulla. (1993). *Modrande och praxis. En feministfilosofisk undersökning.* Göteborg: Daidalos.

Hovelius, Birgitta. (1996). Unga kvinnors hälsoproblem från ungdomsmottagningens perspektiv. In Svenska Läkaresällskapet och Spri. *Tema: Kvinna. Symposier vid Svenska Läkaresällskapets riksstämma 1995* (pp. 111-118). Stockholm: Spris förlag.

Humlesjö, Inger. (1999). Manliga och sega strukturer. *Arbetarhistoria*, 23, (2-3), 21-30.

Håkansson, C., Eklund, M., Lidfeldt, J., Nerbrand, Christina, Samsioe, Göran and Nilsson, P. (2005). Well-being and occupational roles among middle-aged women. *Work*, 24, 341-351.

Härenstam, Annika. (2001). Combining professional work with family responsibilities – a burden or a blessing? *International Journal of Social Science*, 10, 202-214.

Högberg, Ulf. (2013). Personal message to Annika Forssén, 17 April.
Högskoleverket. (2000). Sexuella trakasserier mot studenter: högskolornas åtgärder i Sverige. *Högskoleverkets rapportserie*, 2000, 17 R.
Hölge-Hazelton, Bibi and Malterud, Kirsti. (2009). Gender in medicine – does it matter? *Scandinavian Journal of Public Health*, 37(2), 139-145.
Jacobson, D. (1974). Rejection of the Retiree Role: A Study of Female Industrial Workers in Their 50s. *Human Relations*, 27, 477-492.
Jansson, Christina. (2008). *Maktfyllda möten i medicinska rum: Debatt, kunskap och praktik i svensk förlossningsvård 1960–1985.* [Dissertation.] Lund: Sekel Bokförlag.
Johannisson, Karin. (2001). Gender inequalities in health: An historical and cultural perspective. In Piroska Östlin, Maria Danielsson, Finn Diderichsen, Annika Härenstam and Gudrun Lindberg (eds). *Gender Inequalities in Health* (pp. 99-116). Boston: Harvard University Press.
Jónasdóttir, Anna G. (1991). *Love, Power and Political Interests. Towards a Theory of Patriarchy in Contemporary Western Societies.* [Dissertation.] Örebro: Örebro Studies. University of Örebro.
Jämställdhetsombudsmannen (JämO). (2007). *Handbok om sexuella trakasserier på grund av kön i arbetslivet.* Stockholm: JämO.
Järvholm, Bengt and Reutervall, Christina. (2012). *Arbetsmiljöns bidrag till hjärt-kärlsjukdom. Kunskapsöversikt.* Stockholm: Arbetsmiljöverket/ Swedish Work Environment Authority. Rapport 2012:9.
Karasek, Robert and Theorell, Töres. (1990). *Healthy Work. Stress, Productivity and the Reconstruction of Working Life.* New York: Basic Books.
Kessler, Ronald C. (2003). Epidemiology of women and depression. *Journal of Affective Disorders*, 74, 5-13.
Kitzinger, Sheila. (1992). Birth and violence against women: generating hypotheses from women's accounts of unhappiness after childbirth. In Helen Roberts (ed.). *Women's Health Matters* (pp. 63-80). London: Routledge.
Kofman, Eleonore. (2010). *Gender and International Migration in Europe: Employment, Welfare and Politics.* London: Routledge.
Kvale, Steinar. (1996). *InterViews: An Introduction to Qualitative Research Interviewing* (pp. 160-176). Thousand Oaks, California: Sage Publications.
Lennartsson, Anna-Karin, Theorell, Töres, Rockwell, A., Kushnir, M., and Jonsdottir, I. (2013). Perceived Stress at Work Associated with Lower Levels of DHEA-S. *PloS ONE*, 8(8), e72460.

Lewis, Jerry, Beavers, W. R., Gosset, J. T. and Phillips, V. A. (1976). *No Single Threads: Psychological Health in Family Systems*. New York: Brunner/Mazel Publishers.
Lewis, Charlotte and Mathiassen, Svend E. (2013). *Belastning, genus och hälsa i arbetslivet. Kunskapssammanställning*. Stockholm: Arbetsmiljöverket/ The Swedish Work Environment Authority.
Lindgren, Magnus. (2013). Polisens utredningsverksamhet – ett svek mot våldsdrabbade kvinnor. *Stiftelsen Tryggare Sverige*. http://tryggaresverige.org/polisens-utredningsverksamhet-ett-svek-motvaldsdrabbade-kvinnor
Linn, Gudrun. (1985). *Hur skall badrum byggas för att underlätta städningen?* [Dissertation.] Stockholm: Kungliga tekniska högskolan.
Lundgren, Eva. (1993). *The Process of Normalizing Violence*. Stockholm: ROKS.
Lundgren, Eva, Heimer, Gun, Westerstrand, Jenny and Kalliokoski, Anne-Marie. (2002). *Captured Queen: Men's violence against women in "equal" Sweden – a prevalence study*. Uppsala: Crime Victim Compensation and Support Authority, University of Uppsala. http://sgdatabase.unwomen.org/uploads/Sweden%20-%20Captured%20Queen%20-%20Mens%20violence%20against%20women.pdf
Läkartidningen. (1993). Vetgirig vår på Knistad. Annons. *Läkartidningen*, 90: 88.
Magnusson, Eva. (1997). Talking about gender equality: Swedish women's discourse on the home front. *NORA/Nordic Journal of Feminist and Gender Research*, 5(2), 76-94.
—. (2005). Gendering or Equality in the Lives of Nordic Heterosexual Couples with Children: No Well-paved Avenues Yet. NORA/ Nordic Journal of Feminist and Gender Research, 13(3), 153-163.
—. (2008). The Rhetoric of Inequality: Nordic Women and Men Argue about Sharing House-work. NORA/Nordic Journal of Feminist and Gender Research, 16(2), 79-95.
Main, C., Knight, B., Moxham, T., Gabriel Sanchez, R., Rouqué I Figuls, M. and Bonfill Cosp, X. (2013). Hormone therapy for preventing cardiovascular disease in post-menopausal women. *Cochrane Database Systematic Review* 4.
Malterud, Kirsti. (1993). Strategies for empowering women's voices in the medical culture. *Health Care for Women International*, 14, 365-373.
van Manen, Max. (2002). Care-as-Worry, or "Don't worry, Be happy". *Qualitative Health Research*, 12(2), 262-78.
Mattsson, Karin. (2011). *Varför finns det skillnader i bifallsfrekvensen inom arbetsskadeförsäkringen? En studie om orsaker till skillnader i bifall och avslag mellan kön, födelseland och var beslutet fattas*. Stockholm: Försäkringskassan. Social Insurance Report.

McEwan, Bruce S. and Getz, Linn. (2013). Lifetime experiences, the brain and personalized medicine: an integrative perspective. *Metabolism*, 62(Suppl 1), 20-26.

McPherson, Klim and Hemminki, Elina. (2004). Synthesising licensing data to assess drug safety. *BMJ*, 328, 518-520.

Meinert, C. (1995). The inclusion of women in clinical trials. *Science*, 269, 795-796.

Messing, Karen. (1998). *One-Eyed Science. Occupational Health and Women Workers*. Philadelphia: Temple University Press.

Myrdal, Alva. (1938). Den nyare tidens revolution i kvinnans ställning. In Myrdal, Alva, Andreen, Andrea, Boalt, Karin, Höjer, Signe and Wigforss, Ewa. *Kvinnan, familjen och samhället*. Stockholm: Kooperativa Förbundets Bokförlag.

Myrdal, Alva, Andreen, Andrea, Boalt, Karin, Höjer, Signe and Wigforss, Ewa. (1938). *Kvinnan, familjen och samhället*. Stockholm: Kooperativa Förbundets Bokförlag.

Myrdal, Alva and Myrdal, Gunnar. (1934). *Kris i befolkningsfrågan*. Stockholm: Bonniers Förlag.

Mårtensson, Kristina and Yeshimoch, Wondemeneh. (2013). *Delade turer i välfärdssektorn*. Faktaunderlag till Kommunals kongress i Stockholm 28-31 maj. https://www.kommunal.se/PageFiles/151089/Delade%20turer%20i%20v%C3%A4lf%C3%A4rssektorn%202013%201.6%20minsta%20filstorlek.pdf Accessed 20 Januray 2014.

Nilsen, Ann. (1994). Life-lines – a methodological approach. In Gunilla Bjerén and Inga Elgqvist-Salzman (eds). *Gender and Education in a Life Perspective: Lessons from Scandinavia* (pp. 101-114). Aldershot, UK: Avebury.

Norstedts uppslagsbok. (1962). Stockholm: Norstedts förlag.

Nyberg, Anita. (1987). Vad är förvärvsarbete? *Kvinnovetenskaplig tidskrift*, 8(1), 54-65.

Nyberg, Anita. (1989). *Tekniken – kvinnornas befriare? Hushållsteknik, köpevaror, gifta kvinnors hushållsarbetstid och förvärvsdeltagande, 1930-talet – 1980-talet*. [Dissertation.] Linköping: Linköping Studies in Arts and Science.

Oakley, Anne. (1992). Speech at the 5th International Conference on Women's Health Issues. Copenhagen, Denmark. 26 August.

O'Hara, Michael W. and McCabe, Jennifer E. (2013). Postpartum Depression: Current Status and Future Directions. *Annual Reviews in Clinical Psychology*, 9, 379-407.

Orth-Gomér, Kristina, Moser, Vanja, Blom, May, Wamala, Sara P. and Schenck-Gustafsson, Karin. (1997). Kvinnostress kartläggs: Hjärtsjukdom hos Stockholmskvinnor orsakas i lika hög grad av stress i familjen som i arbetet. *Läkartidningen (Journal of Swedish Medical Association)*, 94(8), 632-638.

Orth-Gomer, Kristina, Wamala, Sarah P., Horsten, M., Schenck-Gustafsson, Karin, Schneiderman, N., and Mittleman, Murray. (2000). Marital stress worsens prognosis in women with coronary heart disease. *JAMA*, 284, 3008-3014.
Phillips, Susan P. (2005). Defining and measuring gender: A social determinant of health whose time has come. *International Journal for Equity in Health*, 4, 11.
——. (2008). Measuring the health effects of gender. *Journal of Epidemiology and Community Health*, 62, 368-371.
Pilver, C. E., Desay, R., Kasl, S. and Levy, B. R. (2011). Lifetime discrimination with greater likelihood of premenstrual dysphoric disorder. *Journal of Women's Health*, 20(6), 923-931.
Pickett, Kate and Wilkinson, Richard. (2009). *The Spirit Level. Why Greater Equality Makes Societies Stronger.* New York: Bloomsbury Press.
Popay, Jennie. (1992). "My health is all right, but I'm just tired all the time": Women's experience of ill health. In Helen Roberts (ed.). *Women's Health Matters* (pp. 99-120). London: Routledge.
Repetti, Rena, Matthews, Karen and Waldron, I. (1989). Employment and Women's Health: Effects of Paid Employment on Women's Mental and Physical Health. *American Psychologist*, 44, 1394-1401.
Risberg, Gunilla. (2004). *"I am solely a professional – neutral and genderless." On gender bias and gender awareness in the medical profession.* [Dissertation.] Umeå: Umeå University, Department of Public Health and Clinical Medicine.
Risberg, Gunilla, Johansson, Eva E., Westman, Göran and Hamberg, Katarina. (2003). Gender in medicine – an issue for women only? A survey of physician teachers' gender attitudes. *International Journal for Equity in Health*, 2, 10.
Riska, Elianne. (2011). Gender and medical career. *Maturitas*, 68, 264-267.
ROKS. Riksorganisationen för kvinnojourer och tjejjourer i Sverige. http://www.roks.se/bestall/bocker-och-skrifterhttp://www.roks.se/about-roks-t
Roos, Eira, Burström, Bo, Saastamoinen, Peppiina and Lahelma, Elina. (2005). A comparative study of the patterning of women's health by family status and employment status in Finland and Sweden. *Social Science & Medicine*, 60, 2443-2451.
Roosouw, J.E., Anderson, G., Prentice, R.L., LaCroix, A.Z., Kooperberg, C. and Stefanick, M.L. (2002). Risks and benefits of estrogen plus progestin in healthy postmenopausal women: principal results from the Women's Health Initiative randomized controlled trial. *JAMA*, 288, 321-333.

Ross, Catherine and Mirowsky, John. (1995). Does Employment Affect Health? *Journal of Health and Social Behavior*, 36, 230-243.
Rostila, Mikael and Toivanen, Susanna. (2012). *Den orättvisa hälsan. Om socioekonomiska skillnader i hälsa och livslängd*. Stockholm: Liber.
Simkin, Penny. (1991). Just another day in a woman's life? Women's long-term perceptions of their first birth experience. Part I. *Birth*, 18, 203-210.
——. (1992). Just another day in a woman's life? Nature and consistency of women's long-term memories of their first birth experience. Part II. *Birth*, 19, 64-81.
Smirthwaite, Goldina. (2007). *(O)jämställdhet i hälsa och vård – en genusmedicinsk kunskapsöversikt*. Stockholm: Svergies kommuner och landsting/ The Swedish Association of Local Authorities and Regions.
Socialstyrelsen/The National Board of Health and Welfare. (1991/2001). Folkhälsorapporten. Stockholm: Socialstyrelsen. http://www.socialstyrelsen.se/
——. (2006). Antidepressiva läkemedel vid psykisk ohälsa. *Studier av praxis i primärvården*, 103-2. http://www.socialstyrelsen.se/
——. (2012). Folkhälsan i Sverige. Årsrapport 2012. http://www.socialstyrelsen.se/
Sommestad, Lena. (1992). Able dairymaids and proficient dairymen: education and de-feminization in the Swedish dairy industry. In *Gender & History*, 4(1), 34-48.
Sorensen, Gloria and Verbrugge, Lois. (1987). Women, work, and health. *Annual Review of Public Health*, 8, 235-251.
SOU (Statens offentliga utredningar). (1938). *Betänkande angående gift kvinnas förvärvsarbete m m*. Kvinnoarbetskommitén.
Spak, Emma and Ålebring, Jonas. (2014). Var tredje underläkare har upplevt sig diskriminerad. *Läkartidningen*, 111(6), 225.
Statistics Sweden. (2003). *Time for everyday life. Women's and men's time use 1990/1991 and 2000/2001. Living conditions*. Report 99.
——. (2012a). *Nu för tiden. En undersökning om svenska folkets tidsanvändning år 2010/11. Living conditions*. Report 123.
——. (2012b). *Women and Men in Sweden. Facts and Figures*. Stockholm: Statistics Sweden.
Ström, Marie. (2014). Upplevd diskriminering vanligt bland läkare. *Läkartidningen*, 111(6), 202.
Studd, John and Nappi, Rosella E. (2012). Reproductive depression. *Gynecological endocrinology: the official journal of the International Society of Gynecological Endocrinology*, 28 (Suppl. 1), 42-45.

Söderquist, J., Wijma, Barbro, Thorbert, G. and Wijma, Klaas. (2009). Risk factors in pregnancy for post-traumatic stress and depression after childbirth. *BJOG/An international Journal of Obstetrics and Gynaecology*, 116, 672-680.

Tesch, Renate. (1990). *Qualitative Research: Analysis Types and Software Tools*. New York: Falmer Press.

Theorell, Töres, Nordemar, Rolf and Michélsen, H. (1993). Pain thresholds during standardized psychological stress in relation to perceived psychosocial work situation. *Journal of Psychosomatic Research*, 37(3), 299-305.

Thompson, Gill and Downe, Sue. (2008). Widening the trauma discourse: The link between childbirth and experiences of abuse. *Journal of Psychosomatic Obstetrics and Gynecology*, 29, 268-273.

Thomsson, Helene. (2013). Kvinnors sjukfrånvaro: En genusanalys. Rapport på uppdrag av Regeringen. Stockholm: Thomsson & Partners AB.

Thorgren, Gunilla. (2011). Ottar och kärleken: En biografi. Stockholm. Norstedts förlag.

Ussher, Jane and Pertz, J. (2013). PMS as a process of negotiation: women's experience and management of premenstrual distress. *Psychological Health*, 28(8), 909-927.

Villar, J., Valladares, E., Wojdyla, D., Zavaleta, N., Carroli, G., Velazco, A. et al. (2006). Caesarean delivery rates and pregnancy outcomes: the 2005 WHO global survey on maternal and perinatal health in Latin America. *Lancet*, 367, 1819-29.

Vingård, Eva and Kilbom, Åsa. (2001). Diseases of the musculoskeletal system and how they affect men and women. In Piroska Östlin, Maria Danielsson, Finn Diderichsen, Annika Härenstam and Gudrun Lindberg (eds). *Gender Inequalities in Health: A Swedish Perspective* (pp. 159-176). Boston: Harvard University Press.

Waldén, Louise. (1990). *Genom symaskinens nålsöga. Teknik och social förändring i kvinnokultur och manskultur*. [Dissertation.] Tema Teknik och social förändring. Universitetet i Linköping. Stockholm: Carlssons förlag.

—. (2001). Female-male, textile-technical: transferring and transforming culture. In *Upholders of Culture: Past and Present: Lectures from an International Seminar Arranged by the Committee on Man, Technology and Society at the Royal Swedish Academy of Engineering Sciences (IVA) in 2000*, 15-23.

Waldenström, Ulla, Hildingsson, Ingegerd, Rubertsson, Christine and Rådestad, Ingela. (2004). A Negative Birth Experience: Prevalence and Risk Factors in a National Sample. *Birth*, 31, 17-27.

Waldron, I., Weiss, C. C. and Hughes, Mary E. (1998). Interacting

Effects of Multiple Roles on Women's Health. *Journal of Health and Social Behavior*, 39, 216-236.

Walters, V. (2004). The Social Context of Women's Health. *BMC Women's Health*, 4 (Suppl. 1), 1-6.

Wennerås, Christina and Wold, Agnes. (1997). Nepotism and sexism in peer-review. *Nature*, 387, 341-343.

WHO. (1992). *Women's Health: Across Age and Frontier*. Geneva: WHO.

Widerström, Karolina. (1924). *Kvinnohygien*. Stockholm: P. A. Norstedt & Söners Förlag.

Wijma, Klaas, Samelius, Lotta, Wingren, Gun and Wijma, Barbro. (2007). The association between ill-health and abuse: a cross-sectional population based study. *Scandinavian Journal of Psychology*, 48, 567-575.

Witkowska, Eva. (2005). Sexual harassment in schools: prevalence, structure and receptions. Stockholm: *Arbetslivsinstitutet*. Serie: Arbete. Hälsa. 2005:10.

Wong, Kathrin. (2010). *Sexual Harassment Around the Globe*. New York: Nova Science Publishers.

Woolf, Virginia. (1929). *A Room of One's Own*. London: Hoghardt Press.

Yee, J. and Schultz, R. (2000). Gender differences in psychiatric morbidity among family caregivers: a review and analysis. *Gerontologist*, 40(2), 147-164.

English-language publications pertaining to this research project

Forssén, Annika and Carlstedt, Gunilla. (2001). Work, Health and Ill Health. New research makes women's experiences visible. *Scandinavian Journal of Primary Health Care*, 19, 154-157.

Forssén, Annika, Carlstedt, Gunilla and Mörtberg, Christina. (2005). Compulsive sensitivity – a consequence of caring: A qualitative investigation into women carers' difficulties in limiting their labours. *Health Care for Women International*, 26, 652-671.

Forssén, Annika and Carlstedt, Gunilla. (2006). "It's heavenly to be alone!": A room of one's own as a health-promoting resource for women. Results from a qualitative study. *Scandinavian Journal of Public Health*, 34, 175-181.

Forssén, Annika. (2007). Humour, beauty and culture as personal health resources – experiences of elderly Swedish women. *Scandinavian Journal of Public Health*, 35, 228-234.

Forssén, Annika and Carlstedt, Gunilla. (2007). Health-promoting Aspects of a Paid Job: Findings in a Qualitative Interview Study With Elderly Women In Sweden. *Health Care for Women International*, 28, 909–929.

Forssén, Annika and Carlstedt, Gunilla. (2008). "You really do something useful with kids." Mothering and Experienced Health and Illness in a Group of Elderly Swedish Women. *Health Care for Women International*, 29, 1019-1039.

Forssén, Annika. (2012). Lifelong Significance of Disempowering Experiences in Prenatal and Maternity Care: Interviews With Elderly Swedish Women. *Qualitative Health Research*, 22(11), 1536-1546.

Lightning Source UK Ltd.
Milton Keynes UK
UKHW022045130920
369846UK00006B/241

9 781860 571442